AF704235

Reconstruction of Facial Skin Defects

Editor

ANTHONY M. BUNNELL

ATLAS OF THE ORAL AND MAXILLOFACIAL SURGERY CLINICS OF NORTH AMERICA

www.oralmaxsurgeryatlas.theclinics.com

Consulting Editor
RUI P. FERNANDES

March 2020 • Volume 28 • Number 1

ELSEVIER

1600 John F. Kennedy Boulevard • Suite 1800 • Philadelphia, Pennsylvania, 19103-2899
http://www.oralmaxsurgeryatlas.theclinics.com

ATLAS OF THE ORAL AND MAXILLOFACIAL SURGERY CLINICS OF NORTH AMERICA Volume 28, Number 1 March 2020 ISSN 1061-3315 ISBN-13: 978-0-323-68334-0

Editor: John Vassallo; j.vassallo@elsevier.com
Developmental Editor: Laura Fisher

© **2020 Elsevier Inc. All rights reserved.**

This periodical and the individual contributions contained in it are protected under copyright by Elsevier, and the following terms and conditions apply to their use:

Photocopying
Single photocopies of single articles may be made for personal use as allowed by national copyright laws. Permission of the Publisher and payment of a fee is required for all other photocopying, including multiple or systematic copying, copying for advertising or promotional purposes, resale, and all forms of document delivery. Special rates are available for educational institutions that wish to make photocopies for non-profit educational classroom use. For information on how to seek permission visit www.elsevier.com/permissions or call: (+44) 1865 843830 (UK)/(+1) 215 239 3804 (USA).

Derivative Works
Subscribers may reproduce tables of contents or prepare lists of articles including abstracts for internal circulation within their institutions. Permission of the Publisher is required for resale or distribution outside the institution. Permission of the Publisher is required for all other derivative works, including compilations and translations (please consult www.elsevier.com/permissions).

Electronic Storage or Usage
Permission of the Publisher is required to store or use electronically any material contained in this periodical, including any article or part of an article (please consult www.elsevier.com/permissions). Except as outlined above, no part of this publication may be reproduced, stored in a retrieval system or transmitted in any form or by any means, electronic, mechanical, photocopying, recording or otherwise, without prior written permission of the Publisher.

Notice
No responsibility is assumed by the Publisher for any injury and/or damage to persons or property as a matter of products liability, negligence or otherwise, or from any use or operation of any methods, products, instructions or ideas contained in the material herein. Because of rapid advances in the medical sciences, in particular, independent verification of diagnoses and drug dosages should be made. Although all advertising material is expected to conform to ethical (medical) standards, inclusion in this publication does not constitute a guarantee or endorsement of the quality or value of such product or of the claims made of it by its manufacturer.

Reprints. For copies of 100 or more of articles in this publication, please contact the Commercial Reprints Department, Elsevier Inc., 360 Park Avenue South, New York, NY 10010-1710. Tel.: 212-633-3874; Fax: 212-633-3820; E-mail: reprints@elsevier.com.

Atlas of the Oral and Maxillofacial Surgery Clinics of North America (ISSN 1061-3315) is published biannually by Elsevier, 360 Park Avenue South, New York, NY 10010-1710. Months of issue are March and September. Periodicals postage paid at New York, NY and additional mailing offices. Subscription prices are $469.00 for international individual, $396.00 for US individual, $416.00 for Canadian individual; $220.00 for international student, $100.00 for US student and Canadian student; $583.00 for international institution, $583.00 for Canadian institution, $475.00 for US institution. Foreign air speed delivery is included in all *Clinics* subscription prices. All prices are subject to change without notice. POSTMASTER: Send address changes to *Atlas of the Oral and Maxillofacial Surgery Clinics of North America*, Health Sciences Division, Subscription Customer Service, 3251 Riverport Lane, Maryland Heights, MO 63043. Tel: 1-800-654-2452 (U.S. and Canada); 314-447-8871 (outside U.S. and Canada). Fax: 314-417-8029. E-mail: journalscustomerservice-usa@elsevier.com (for print support); journalsonline support-usa@elsevier.com (for online support).

Atlas of the Oral and Maxillofacial Surgery Clinics of North America is covered in *MEDLINE/PubMed (Index Medicus)*.

Printed in the United States of America.

Contributors

CONSULTING EDITOR

RUI P. FERNANDES, MD, DMD, FACS, FRCS(Ed)
Clinical Professor and Chief, Division of Head and Neck Surgery, Program Director, Head and Neck Oncologic Surgery and Microvascular Reconstruction Fellowship, Departments of Oral and Maxillofacial Surgery, Neurosurgery, and Orthopaedic Surgery and Rehabilitation, University of Florida Health Science Center, University of Florida College of Medicine–Jacksonville, Jacksonville, Florida

EDITOR

ANTHONY M. BUNNELL, MD, DMD, FACS
Assistant Professor, Division of Head and Neck Surgery, Department of Oral and Maxillofacial Surgery, University of Florida College of Medicine–Jacksonville, Jacksonville, Florida

AUTHORS

AL HAITHAM AL SHETAWI, MD, DMD, FACS
Division of Surgical Oncology, Department of Surgery, Vassar Brother Medical Center, Nuvance Health, Dyson Center for Cancer Care, Poughkeepsie, New York

KEVIN ARCE, MD, DMD
Division Chair and Assistant Professor of Surgery, Section of Head and Neck Oncologic Surgery and Reconstruction, Division of Oral and Maxillofacial Surgery, Department of Surgery, Mayo Clinic, Mayo College of Medicine, Rochester, Minnesota

HANS C. BROCKHOFF II, DDS, MD
Assistant Professor, Department of Surgery, Texas Tech University Health Sciences Center El Paso, El Paso, Texas

ANTHONY M. BUNNELL, MD, DMD, FACS
Assistant Professor, Division of Head and Neck Surgery, Department of Oral and Maxillofacial Surgery, University of Florida College of Medicine–Jacksonville, Jacksonville, Florida

SRINIVASA RAMA CHANDRA, MD, BDS, FDSRCS(Eng), FIBCSOMS (Onc- Recon), FACS
Plastic Surgery Resident, Division of Plastic and Reconstruction Surgery, Department of Surgery, University of Nebraska Medical Center, Division of OMFS–Head and Neck Surgery, Head and Neck Oncology and Microvascular Reconstructive Surgery, Assistant Professor, Department of Surgery, University of Nebraska Medical Center, Fred & Pamela Buffett Cancer Center, Omaha, Nebraska

ALLEN CHENG, MD, DDS, FACS
Consultant and Medical Director, The Head and Neck Institute, Head and Neck Surgical Associates, Attending Surgeon, Providence Cancer Institute, Medical Director, Oral, Head and Neck Cancer Program, Legacy Cancer Institute, Portland, Oregon

KYLE S. ETTINGER, MD, DDS
Assistant Professor of Surgery, Section of Head and Neck Oncologic Surgery and Reconstruction, Division of Oral and Maxillofacial Surgery, Department of Surgery, Mayo Clinic, Mayo College of Medicine, Rochester, Minnesota

Contributors

RUI P. FERNANDES, MD, DMD, FACS, FRCS(Ed)
Clinical Professor and Chief, Division of Head and Neck Surgery, Program Director, Head and Neck Oncologic Surgery and Microvascular Reconstruction Fellowship, Departments of Oral and Maxillofacial Surgery, Neurosurgery, and Orthopaedic Surgery and Rehabilitation, University of Florida Health Science Center, University of Florida College of Medicine—Jacksonville, Jacksonville, Florida

DANIEL HAMMER, DDS
Fellow, Division of Maxillofacial Oncology and Reconstructive Surgery, Department of Oral and Maxillofacial Surgery, John Peter Smith Hospital, Fort Worth, Texas

HEIDI H. HON, MD
Plastic Surgery Resident, Division of Plastic and Reconstruction Surgery, Department of Surgery, University of Nebraska Medical Center, Division of OMFS—Head and Neck Surgery, Head and Neck Oncology and Microvascular Reconstructive Surgery, Assistant Professor, Department of Surgery, University of Nebraska Medical Center, Fred & Pamela Buffett Cancer Center, Omaha, Nebraska

RODERICK KIM, DDS, MD
Assistant Fellowship Director, Director of Research, Division of Maxillofacial Oncology and Reconstructive Surgery, Department of Oral and Maxillofacial Surgery, John Peter Smith Hospital, Fort Worth, Texas

MAREK OGLEDZKI, DMD, MD
Head and Neck Oncologic and Microvascular Reconstructive Surgery Fellow, Ascension-St. John Hospital, Warren, Michigan

ASHISH A. PATEL, MD, DDS, FACS
Consultant and Director of Microvascular Surgery, The Head and Neck Institute, Head and Neck Surgical Associates, Medical Director, Cranio-Oral and Maxillofacial and Neck Trauma, Legacy Emanuel Medical Center, Attending Surgeon, Providence Cancer Institute, Portland, Oregon

DANIEL PETRISOR, DMD, MD, FACS
Assistant Professor and Director, Head and Neck Oncologic and Microvascular Reconstructive Surgery, Department of Oral and Maxillofacial Surgery, Oregon Health & Science University, Mark O. Hatfield Research Center, Portland, Oregon

CARLOS A. RAMIREZ, MD, DDS
Fellowship Director, Head and Neck Oncology/Microvascular Surgery, Chief and Program Director, Oral/Maxillofacial Surgery, Assistant Professor, Michigan State University, East Lansing, Michigan; Director, Microvascular Surgery, Ascension-St. John Hospital, Detroit, Michigan

ALBA SANJUAN-SANJUAN, MD
Oral and Maxillofacial Surgeon, Ascension-St. John Hospital, Warren, Michigan

WILLIAM WALSH THOMAS, MD
Microvascular Fellow, Oregon Health & Science University, Portland, Oregon

CONG VO, DDS, MD
Oral and Maxillofacial Surgery Resident, Oregon Health & Science University, Mark O. Hatfield Research Center, Portland, Oregon

FAYETTE WILLIAMS, DDS, MD, FACS
Division and Fellowship Director, Division of Maxillofacial Oncology and Reconstructive Surgery, Department of Oral and Maxillofacial Surgery, John Peter Smith Hospital, Fort Worth, Texas

Contents

Glabellar Flaps for Reconstruction of Skin Defects 43

Alba Sanjuan-Sanjuan, Marek Ogledzki, and Carlos A. Ramirez

Bilobed Flaps 49

Cong Vo, William Walsh Thomas, Hans C. Brockhoff II, and Daniel Petrisor

ATLAS OF THE ORAL AND MAXILLOFACIAL SURGERY CLINICS OF NORTH AMERICA

FORTHCOMING ISSUES

September 2020

Computer Aided Oral and Maxillofacial Surgery
Kevin Arce, *Editor*

March 2021

Orbital Surgery
Leander Dubois and A.G. (Eddy) Becking, *Editors*

PREVIOUS ISSUES

September 2019

Trauma Surgery
Alaaaldin M. Radwan and Robert A. Strauss, *Editors*

March 2019

Sleep Surgery
Stanley Yung-Chuan Liu, *Editor*

SERIES OF RELATED INTEREST

Oral and Maxillofacial Surgery Clinics
http://www.oralmaxsurgery.theclinics.com/

Dental Clinics
http://www.dental.theclinics.com

THE CLINICS ARE NOW AVAILABLE ONLINE!

Access your subscription at:
www.theclinics.com

Preface

The Facial Skin Defect: A Reconstructive Opportunity

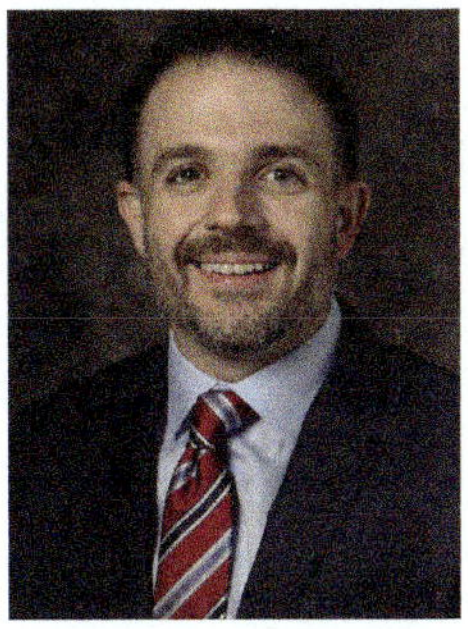

Anthony M. Bunnell, MD, DMD, FACS
Editor

I am honored and grateful for the opportunity to introduce this issue of the *Atlas of the Oral and Maxillofacial Surgery Clinics of North America* devoted to reconstruction of facial skin defects. Each day, the maxillofacial surgeon is faced with many challenges and options in reconstructing facial skin defects. The key is to select the most appropriate reconstructive method and setting for this to take place. This may be a daunting task, but when equipped with the proper tools, a reconstructive challenge can turn into an opportunity to produce an aesthetically pleasing reconstructive outcome. The goal of this issue of the *Atlas of the Oral and Maxillofacial Surgery Clinics of North America* is to provide the tools necessary for the reader to develop a surgical armamentarium of the most commonly used local flaps in facial reconstruction.

The reader will find that each article within this *Atlas of the Oral and Maxillofacial Surgery Clinics of North America* is dedicated to a single flap for an in-depth review of flap design and execution. Pertinent surgical anatomy as well as a "how-to" explanation of flap elevation is incorporated into each article to provide the reader a comprehensive understanding on each flap described. The authors have also offered their expertise by sharing clinical applications through case examples as well as surgical pearls and pitfalls one may encounter during the reconstructive process.

I would be remiss if I did not acknowledge the hard work and dedication of the authors in order to produce this *Atlas of the Oral and Maxillofacial Surgery Clinics of North America*. It has been a great privilege to work with these authors, and I express my gratitude for their time and contributions in producing these informative articles. Thank you to Dr. Rui Fernandes, the Consulting Editor, for his guidance and support of this project. I also want to thank my mentors, colleagues, fellows, and residents at the University of Florida, who continue to inspire me to be a better surgeon and teacher each day. Lastly, I want to acknowledge the endless support from my family in allowing me to pursue this endeavor.

It is my hope that the readers will find this *Atlas of the Oral and Maxillofacial Surgery Clinics of North America* a useful tool in facial reconstruction and will provide their patients the *best reconstructive outcome*.

Anthony M. Bunnell, MD, DMD, FACS
Division of Head and Neck Surgery
Department of Oral and Maxillofacial Surgery
University of Florida College of Medicine–Jacksonville
653-1 West 8th Street
Jacksonville, FL 32209, USA

E-mail address:
anthony.bunnell@jax.ufl.edu

Atlas Oral Maxillofacial Surg Clin N Am 28 (2020) ix
1061-3315/20/© 2019 Published by Elsevier Inc.
https://doi.org/10.1016/j.cxom.2019.12.001

The Facial Skin Defect

Preop to Postop

Anthony M. Bunnell, MD, DMD

KEYWORDS

• Facial reconstruction • Nasal reconstruction • Cheek reconstruction • Local flap • Pedicled flap • Mohs reconstruction

KEY POINTS

- Reconstruction of facial skin defects regardless of cause has important psychosocial implications, and multiple factors must be considered when choosing the final reconstructive plan.
- Photography is an invaluable tool for the surgeon during all phases of reconstruction regardless of level of experience.
- Immediate or delayed reconstruction following ablation of skin cancer each has its own advantages and disadvantages. The surgeon must be flexible when deciding the most optimal setting for the reconstruction to take place.
- The subunit principle remains an important guide for reconstructing facial defects.

Introduction

Skin cancers are the most common types of cancer with approximately 5.4 million basal cell and squamous cell skin cancers diagnosed each year in the United States. These cancers affect approximately 3.3 million Americans each year, as some people are often diagnosed with more than one skin malignancy. Eight out of ten are basal cell carcinomas, with squamous cell carcinoma occurring less often.[1] The high incidence of cutaneous squamous cell carcinoma and basal cell carcinoma has been shown to be related to sun exposure and mutagenic effects. Other risk factors for developing nonmelanoma skin cancer include immunosuppression, male gender, and advanced age. With the steadily increasing population of the elderly population in the United States, the need for removal of these facial skin lesions and reconstruction of the associated defect continues to be in high demand. Because of the location of these lesions, patients are frequently concerned regarding the esthetic outcome following the procedure. Multiple studies have demonstrated that skin tumors located on the face and facial scarring are associated with significant psychological morbidity.[2–4] The concerns regarding scarring have been shown to have an impact on quality of life.[3,5–8] Reconstruction of these facial skin defects can be a challenging but rewarding experience for both the patient and reconstructive surgeon. When planning for reconstruction, one must consider tumor characteristics, defect location and size, aesthetic considerations, and patient comorbidities. Including these factors in the process of evaluating the skin defect will provide an optimal reconstructive outcome.

Department of Oral and Maxillofacial Surgery, University of Florida College of Medicine-Jacksonville, 653-1 West 8th Street, Jacksonville, FL 32209, USA
E-mail address: Anthony.bunnell@jax.ufl.edu

Atlas Oral Maxillofacial Surg Clin N Am 28 (2020) 1-5
1061-3315/20/Published by Elsevier Inc.
https://doi.org/10.1016/j.cxom.2019.11.006

Preoperative planning

Anesthetic evaluation

Patients presenting for reconstruction of their facial defect may undergo the procedure in a variety of settings. These procedures can take place in the office, sedation suite, or operating room. Reconstruction can take place under local anesthesia, local anesthesia with sedation, monitored anesthesia care, or general anesthesia with endotracheal intubation. This will depend on patient factors, including NPO status, comorbidities, location of the defect, and complexity of the reconstruction. The setting that this takes place offers its own advantages and disadvantages and must be tailored to each patient. Minor procedures that take place under local anesthesia with sedation are convenient for both the patient and the surgeon. In-office procedures offer the advantage for those patients who present to the office for reconstruction following a Mohs procedure. These patients are often added onto the schedule later in the day making in-office procedures easier to schedule than trying to "add-on" an operating room case late in the day. These same patients, however, may have a complex medical history that may warrant a general anesthetic and may need to be delayed for reconstruction. The reconstruction plan may also change following the ablative procedure. The defect may be larger than the surgeon anticipates and the reconstruction plan may change from a single stage flap to a multi stage paramedian flap with cartilage grafting. The reconstructive surgeon must keep this in mind when coordinating schedules and preparing to take the patient to the operating room. The patient must also be made aware of these possibilities and prepared to undergo a delayed reconstruction the following day if necessary. The advantages and disadvantages to delayed reconstruction are discussed elsewhere in this article.

Clinical photography

"A picture is worth a thousand words." This adage suggests that complex or multiple ideas can be conveyed by a single image and has clinical significance in all stages of facial reconstruction. Photos assist with clinical documentation in the preoperative, intraoperative, and postoperative settings. Photos should include not only the defect or anatomic subunit but also the entire face in multiple views. This will also be helpful in evaluation for potential flap donor sites when considering local versus regional flap reconstruction (Fig. 1 A, B). These images are invaluable to the surgeon, regardless of the level of experience. For the novice surgeon, pictures assist with developing treatment plans. As the surgeon builds their practice and develops a photo database, this provides instant feedback on surgical outcomes. When planning treatment for a complex or multifacial subunit defect, the surgeon is often left with personal experience to plan for the most appropriate reconstruction.[9] Developing a personal photographic library of surgical cases will assist with treatment planning for future complex cases. For the academic surgeon, these photos are also invaluable for resident training. These photos can assist with education, developing a treatment plan, and providing feedback. Server-based photographic databases now exist to assist with photo storage and organization and will help with self-review and assessment for all levels of experience.[9]

Immediate versus delayed reconstruction

Facial skin defects are often created and reconstructed on the same day. There are situations in which the reconstruction may not occur simultaneously. This is most common when the ablation occurs with a Mohs surgeon. There are many reasons reconstruction can be delayed from the time of initial resection, which includes coordinating of schedules, operating room, or clinic availability. Time to reconstruction has been reported in the literature to range from 1 day to more than 1 month.[10–12] There are benefits but also pitfalls to delaying reconstruction. Delaying reconstruction offers increased time for surgical planning, patient counseling, and contemplation as well as increased blood supply to the cauterized wound bed.[10] There are obvious disadvantages associated with delayed reconstruction including patient satisfaction. The biggest question in regard to delayed reconstruction includes the perceived increased risk of infection with an "open wound" from the time of resection to reconstruction. The literature is variable on the timing of reconstruction. Miller and colleagues[10] reported no association between timing of Mohs reconstructive surgery and complications including infection, dehiscence, and partial or full graft or flap loss. Patel and colleagues[12] showed in their study that delaying reconstruction for more than 2 days was associated with a higher rate of complications. Patel's group also showed that smoking status, wound size, full-thickness defects, composite grafts, and interposition flaps with cartilage grafts were associated with a higher rate of complications. As expected, multiple studies have shown that smoking is associated with higher rates. Counseling the patient on the effects of delayed healing due to tobacco use and counseling on smoking cessation is essential. Regardless of the timing of reconstruction, communication with the patient about the timing of reconstruction and expectations will improve patient satisfaction.

Surgical technique

Intraoperative planning

Reconstruction can range from a simple primary closure to a complex reconstruction requiring multistage procedures and cartilage grafts. Fortunately most defects can be reconstructed in a single stage using one of the many local flaps discussed elsewhere in this atlas. The key is to determine

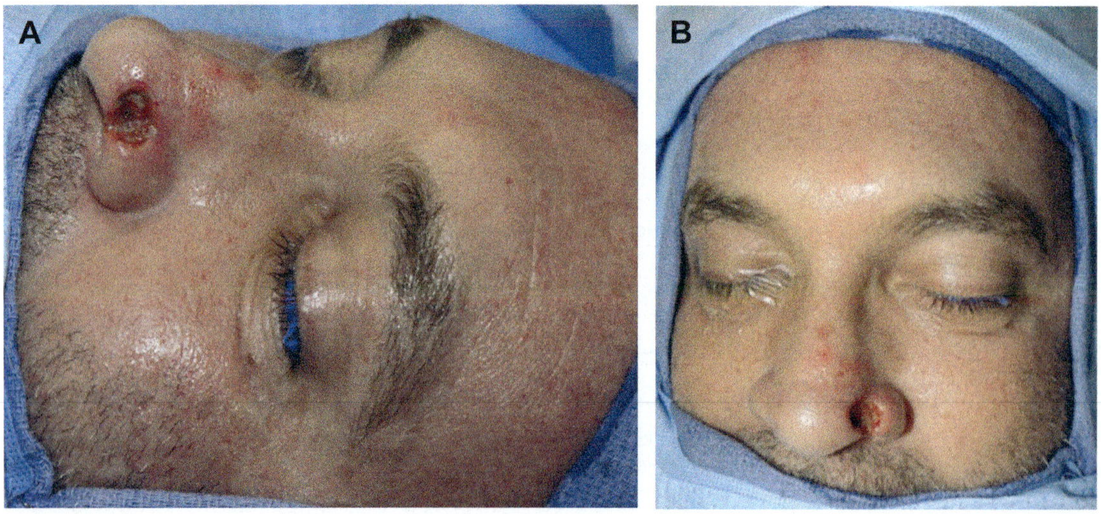

Fig. 1 Intraoperative frontal view of nasal skin defect following Mohs procedure. (*A*) Oblique view including entire mid and upper face within field to include possible flap donor sites. (*B*) Clinical photos should be taken in a consistent replicable fashion each time to build a photo "library" of cases that may assist with future treatment planning.

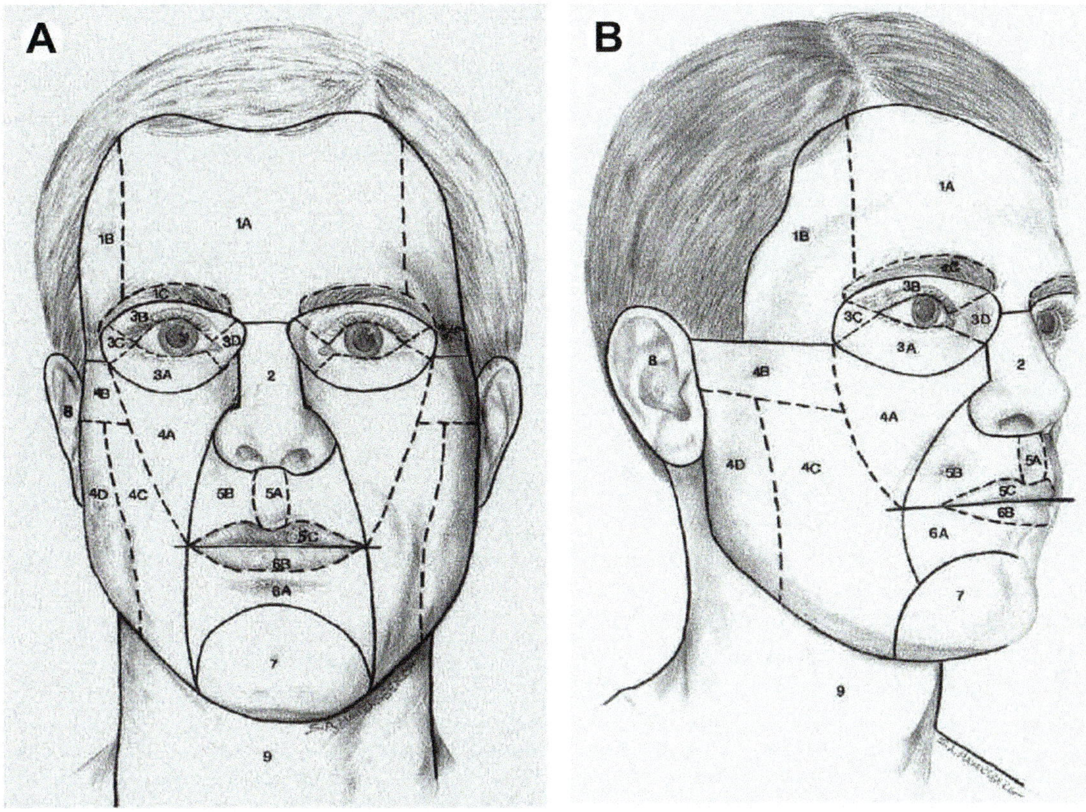

Fig. 2 Frontal (*A*) and Profile (*B*) view of the units and subunits of the face for facial reconstruction. 1, Forehead unit (1A, central subunit; 1B, lateral subunit; 1C, eyebrow subunit); 2, nasal unit; 3, eye lid units (3A, lower lid unit; 3B, upper lid unit; 3C, lateral canthal subunit; 3D, medial canthal subunit); 4, cheek unit (4A, medial subunit; 4B, zygomatic subunit; 4C, lateral subunit; 4D, buccal subunit); 5, upper lip unit (5A, philtrum subunit; 5B, lateral subunit; 5C, mucosal subunit); 6, lower lip unit (6A, central subunit; 6B, mucosal subunit); 7, mental unit; 8, auricular unit; 9, neck unit. (*From* Fattahi TT. An overview of facial aesthetic units. J Oral Maxillofac Surg. 2003;61(10):1208; with permission.)

which flap is suitable not only for the defect but also meets the needs of each patient. Patient's self-identity and perception are greatly influenced by a surgeon's manipulation and handling of facial tissues.[13] When evaluating the defect, it is important to use the facial subunit principle as a guide to plan the final reconstruction. Regional aesthetic units of the face were first described by Gonzales-Ulloa to highlight the need for restoring facial skin units in complete regions. Burget and Menick[14,15] then went on to incorporate principles of psychology and visual perceptions into surgical technique and introduced the concept of the subunit theory (Fig. 2). Menick describes the concave and convex surfaces of the face that allow for different light reflections. Menick also reported that when suture lines and grafts are placed in a particular subunit, the natural appearance of lights and shadows is reestablished preventing them from being easily noticed to the untrained

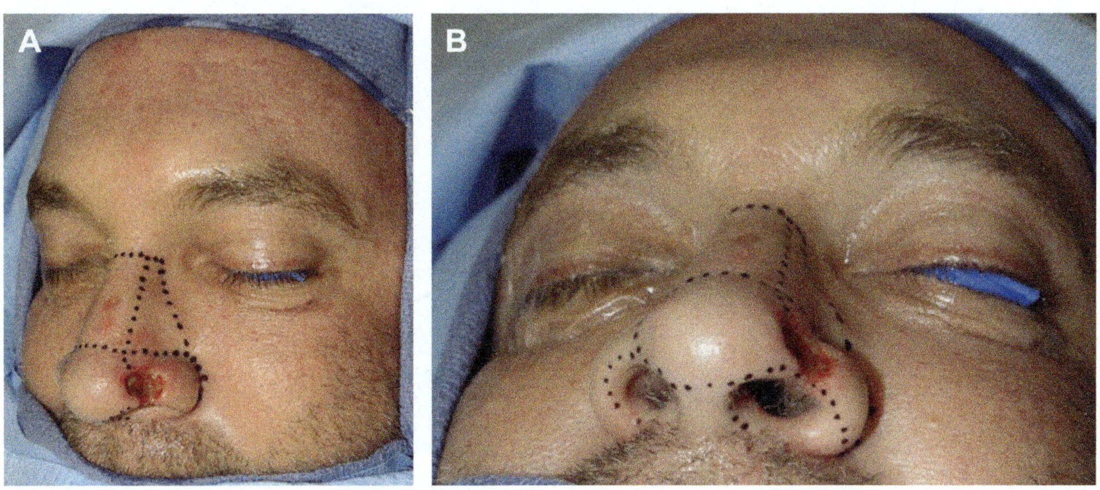

Fig. 3 (*A*) Nasal Ala defect with Nasal Subunits outlined prior to reconstruction. (*B*) Outlining nasal subunits allows the surgeon to assess the size and thickness of the defect in relation to the subunits involved.

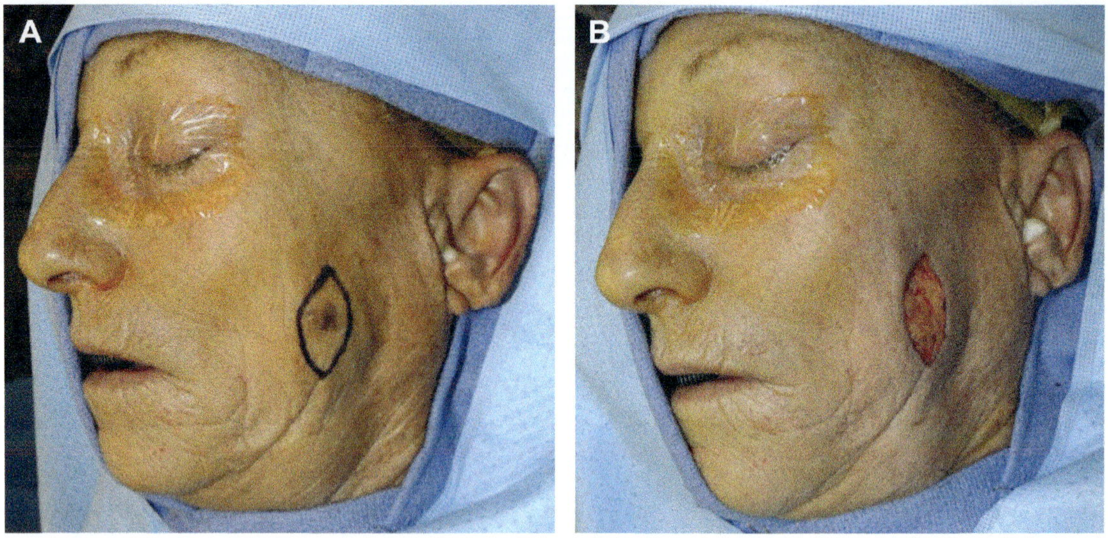

Fig. 4 (*A*) Intraoperative view of planned resection with appropriate oncologic margins. (*B*) Incorporating incisions within resting skin tension lines (RSTLs) facilitates an aesthetic closure.

eye. Burget and Menick's nasal subunit principle states that when a defect of the nose covers greater than 50% of a subunit, the remaining subunit is excised and the entire subunit is repaired. Although some studies have reviewed less or more aggressive approaches to the subunit principle,[16–18] a recent report on trends in nasal reconstruction by Larrabee and colleagues showed that most of the surgeons continue to use the subunit principle for reconstructing large defects of the nasal tip and ala, whereas a modified subunit approach is taken by many surgeons to reconstruct nasal dorsum and sidewall subunits.[19] Regardless of the approach toward reconstruction, thorough understanding of the facial subunits is helpful in planning for both the ablative and reconstructive process (Fig. 3 A, B). Placing incisions and flap margins within resting skin tension lines or along borders of facial subunits allows the surgeon to camouflage flap into the appearance of normal anatomic features (Fig. 4 A, B). These principles serve as a foundation for local flap reconstruction and assist the surgeon when developing the final reconstructive plan.

Postoperative considerations

Patients are seen for initial postoperative visit within the first week to evaluate healing and overall wound care. Sutures can be selectively removed depending on flap type, location, and surgeon preference. Wound care is again reviewed with the patient. Bacitracin/polymyxin B antibiotic ointment is recommended in the immediate post operative period but prolonged use is discouraged. Judicious use of antibiotic ointment is recommended as to not interfere with wound healing. The patient is seen again the following week to remove any remaining sutures (if intentionally left in place) and initial postoperative photos are taken (Fig. 5 A, B). Another set of photos is then taken when the patient is seen at 3-month follow-up visit. Discussion with patient includes their feedback on reconstructive outcome and wishes for any further adjunctive procedures (scar revision, flap debulking, etc) (Fig. 5C). As mentioned previously, the use of photos can be helpful in educating the patient on their expected course

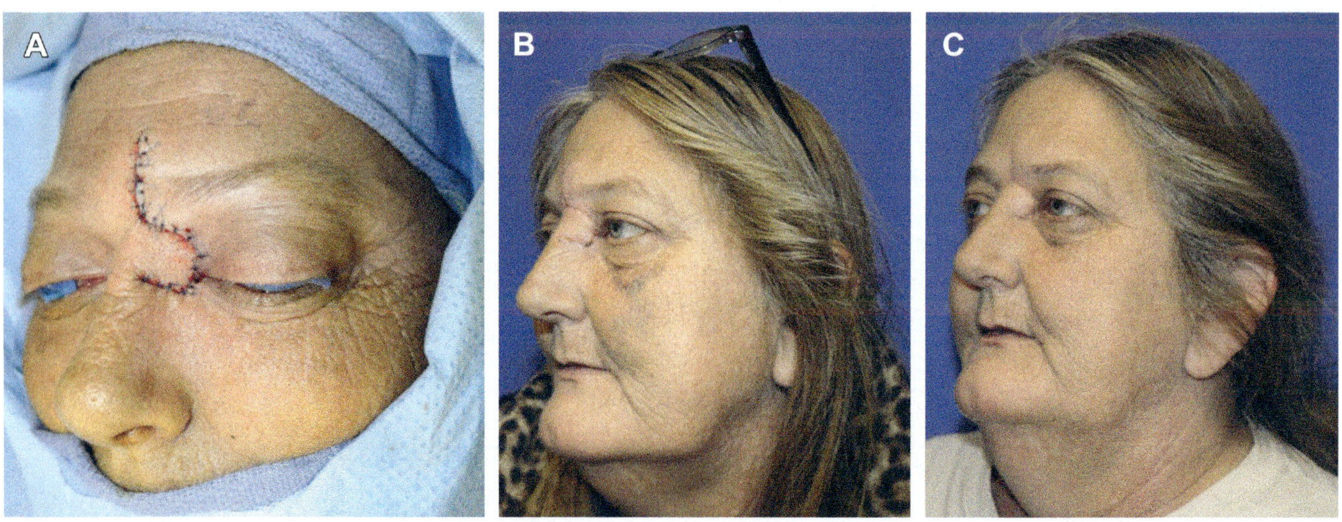

Fig. 5 (*A*) Intraoperative view following glabellar reconstruction of medial canthal defect following resection of basal cell carcinoma. (*B*) Early post operative view two weeks following reconstruction with glabellar flap. (*C*) Three month post operative view to assess for any needed scar revision, flap debulking or other adjunctive procedures.

and patient satisfaction on their outcome (Figs. 2–5). Complication rates for reconstruction of facial defects have been reported in the literature ranging from 1% to 19%.[9,10,12,20–22] Complications related to bleeding and infection are the most common complications reported in the literature. Complications or adverse outcomes can be stratified into different groups based on patent factors, anatomic location, and reconstruction method. Complications include hemorrhage, hematoma, wound infection, flap necrosis, and dehiscence. Anatomic location–based complications include telecanthus, epiphora, eyelid retraction, notching, and nasal vestibular stenosis. Patient factors such as smoking status, comorbidities including diabetes, the use of anticoagulant, and patient compliance will influence wound healing and must be taken into consideration when planning the final reconstruction.

Disclosure

The author has nothing to disclose.

References

1. Siegel RL, Miller KD, Jemal A. Cancer statistics, 2019. CA Cancer J Clin 2019;69:7.
2. Dropkin MJ. Body image and quality of life after head and neck cancer surgery. CancerPract 1999;7:309.
3. Lee EH, Klassen AF, Cano SJ, et al. FACE-Q Skin Cancer Module for measuring patient-reported outcomes following facial skin cancer surgery. Br J Dermatol 2018;179:88.
4. Steinbauer J, Koller M, Kohl E, et al. Quality of life in health care of non-melanoma skin cancer - results of a pilot study. J DtschDermatolGes 2011;9:129.
5. Dey JK, Ishii LE, Joseph AW, et al. The cost of facial deformity: a health utility and valuation study. JAMAFacialPlastSurg 2016;18:241.
6. Dey JK, Ishii LE, Byrne PJ, et al. The social penalty of facial lesions: new evidence supporting high-quality reconstruction. JAMA Facial Plast Surg 2015;17:90.
7. Godoy A, Ishii M, Byrne PJ, et al. How facial lesions impact attractiveness and perception: differential effects of size and location. Laryngoscope 2011;121:2542.
8. Burdon-Jones D, Thomas P, Baker R. Quality of life issues in non-metastatic skin cancer. Br J Dermatol 2010;162:147.
9. Miller MQ, Rikhi SR, Park SS, et al. An innovative photographic database for cutaneous facial defects. Laryngoscope 2016;126:2451.
10. Miller MQ, David AP, McLean JE, et al. Christophel J: Association of Mohs reconstructive surgery timing with postoperative complications. JAMA Facial Plast Surg 2018;20:122.
11. David AP, Miller MQ, Park SS, et al. Comparison of outcomes of early vs delayed graft reconstruction of Mohsmicrographic surgery defects. JAMA Facial Plast Surg 2019;21:89.
12. Patel SA, Liu JJ, Murakami CS, et al. Complication rates in delayed reconstruction of the head and neck after Mohsmicrographic surgery. JAMA Facial Plast Surg 2016;18:340.
13. Fattahi TT. An overview of facial aesthetic units. J Oral MaxillofacSurg 2003;61:1207.
14. Burget GC, Menick FJ. The subunit principle in nasal reconstruction. Plast Reconstr Surg 1985;76:239.
15. Menick FJ. Defects of the nose, lip, and cheek: rebuilding the composite defect. Plast Reconstr Surg 2007;120:887.
16. Shumrick KA, Campbell A, Becker FF, et al. Modification of the subunit principle for reconstruction of nasal tip and dorsum defects. Arch Facial Plast Surg 1999;1:9.
17. Rohrich RJ, Griffin JR, Ansari M, et al. Nasal reconstruction-beyond aesthetic subunits: a 15-year review of 1334 cases. Plast Reconstr Surg 2004;114:1405.
18. Haugen TW, Frodel JL. Reconstruction of complex nasal dorsal and sidewall defects: is the nasal sidewall subunit necessary? Arch Facial Plast Surg 2011;13:343.
19. Larrabee YC, Phillips DJ, Sclafani AP. Trends in nasal subunit reconstruction by facial plastic and reconstructive surgeons. Facial Plast Surg 2017;33:17.
20. Berens AM, Akkina SR, Patel SA. Complications in facial Mohs defect reconstruction. Curr Opin Otolaryngol Head Neck Surg 2017;25:258.
21. Sclafani AP, Sclafani JA, Sclafani AM. Successes, revisions, and postoperative complications in 446 Mohs defect repairs. Facial PlastSurg 2012;28:358.
22. Egeler SA, Johnson AR, Ibrahim AMS, et al. Reconstruction of Mohs defects located in the head and neck. J Craniofac Surg 2019;30:412.

The Nasolabial Flap

Ashish A. Patel, MD, DDS [a,b,c,*], Allen Cheng, MD, DDS [a,c,d]

KEYWORDS

• Nasolabial flap • Facial reconstruction • Skin flaps • Local flap • Nasal reconstruction • Oral reconstruction

KEY POINTS

- This article highlights the history, applications, and versatility of the nasolabial flap.
- Variations of flap design, harvest, and inset are described.
- The reader is presented with 5 patient examples using the nasolabial flap for maxillofacial reconstruction.

Introduction

The nasolabial flap has been commonly described and used for facial soft tissue reconstruction since the 19th century. However, the first recorded description dates back to an Indian surgeon, Sushruta, in 600 BCE. The ease of harvest, robust blood supply, and versatility of the flap lends itself to multiple applications. When based axially, it can be carried on the facial artery as an inferiorly based flap, or angular artery as a superiorly based flap. For most applications on the face, random pattern harvest is favorable and allows a thinner, more pliable flap to match the recipient site soft tissue.

Anatomy

The nasolabial region anatomy is surprisingly more complex than it seems. The nasolabial crease runs linearly from 1 cm superior and just lateral to the ala of the nose to 1 cm lateral to the oral commissure. Several reports and anatomic studies have demonstrated the presence of muscle fibers from the zygomaticus major that insert in the dermis of this crease.[1] The vascular supply of this region is derived from perforating branches of the facial artery inferiorly, and angular artery superiorly. This flap is most commonly harvested without its underlying named vessel to maintain thinness, although axial pattern flaps can extend length considerably. The nasolabial crease serves as the major anatomic marker for linear orientation of the flap.

[a] The Head and Neck Institute, Head and Neck Surgical Associates, 1849 Northwest Kearney Street, Suite 300, Portland, OR 97209, USA
[b] Cranio-Oral and Maxillofacial and Neck Trauma, Legacy Emanuel Medical Center, 2801 N. Gantenbein Avenue, Portland OR 97227, USA
[c] Providence Cancer Institute, 4805 NE Glisan Street, Suite 11N-7, Portland, OR 97213, USA
[d] Oral, Head and Neck Cancer Program, Legacy Cancer Institute, 1130 NW 22nd Avenue, Portland, OR 97210, USA
* Corresponding author. The Head and Neck Institute, Head and Neck Surgical Associates, 1849 Northwest Kearney Street, Suite 300, Portland, OR 97209.
E-mail address: patela@head-neck.com
Twitter: @PatelMDDDS (A.A.P.); @Head_NeckSurg (A.C.)

Preoperative planning

The nasolabial flap may be used as a random or axial pattern flap and can be pedicled superiorly or inferiorly. Preoperative history and physical examination is critical in determining the flap variant to be used. Prior facial incisions, scars, and local flap harvest sites may preclude its use if the subdermal vascular plexus has been disturbed. Previous surgery, neck dissection, and/or radiation therapy resulting in facial or angular artery compromise may limit the use of axial pattern flaps or extended flaps. There are several reports of successful standard random pattern nasolabial flaps in patients with concomitant ipsilateral radial neck dissection and facial artery sacrifice.

A pinch test can be used to assess flap width to be harvested starting 2 to 3 mm lateral to the nasolabial crease extending laterally into the cheek. The optimal width of the base of the flap should be approximately 2 cm. This ensures adequate capture of the subdermal vascular plexus and associated perforators, but any wider may limit the arc of rotation. The length of the flap should be within the boundaries of the nasolabial fold for acceptable donor site closure. It is important to limit width medial to the medial canthus to prevent eyelid distortion during donor site closure. In excessively long flaps, the perfusion pressure to the distal aspect may not be adequate for viability. This point is particularly important when harvesting a thin flap that does not include the named axial vessel.[2]

A suture or unfolded surgical sponge may be used to design the overall dimensions of the flap. Gauze or suture is used to simulate the flap length and rotated around the proposed base to determine its reach into the recipient site. Adequate length should be incorporated to allow for a tension-free inset. The arc of rotation can exceed 90° with careful undermining around the base of flap.

Surgical approach

After marking as outlined, harvest of the flap commences by completing the skin incisions while maintaining the base of the flap wider than its distal extension. A distal to proximal harvest with monopolar cautery or a scalpel can be completed expeditiously within the subcutaneous fat. Care

Atlas Oral Maxillofacial Surg Clin N Am 28 (2020) 7-12
1061-3315/20/© 2019 Elsevier Inc. All rights reserved.
https://doi.org/10.1016/j.cxom.2019.10.002

should be taken to not disrupt the muscles of facial expression and stay superficial to the superficial musculoaponeurotic system (SMAS). Because the distal one-third to one-half of the flap will most likely be used for the planned reconstruction, maintaining the desired thickness is critical. A thick, but narrow flap is difficult to inset because the recipient bed (facial skin, intraoral mucosa) will be considerably thinner. This offset in thickness can result in tenting of the flap and internal compression when insetting, leading to venous obstruction. Maintaining a thin layer of subcutaneous fat distally ensures random pattern subdermal plexus capture, while allowing appropriate thickness match for reconstruction.

As the dissection proceeds proximally, the flap harvest may be completed in a deeper plane. Including the angular or facial vessels; however, necessitates dissection in a supraperiosteal plane, which is generally not required. It is important to avoid the temptation to back-cut the base of the flap to increase rotational arc or avoid a standing cutaneous cone as this will compromise the vascularity of the distal third.

Donor site closure

Because the donor site is central on the face, a meticulous tension-free closure is required to prevent unfavorable scarring or facial distortion. Skin flaps should be sharply raised in a supra-SMAS plane, taking care to raise more length laterally than medially. This maneuver is best accomplished with facelift or Dean's scissors. Once the flaps can be closed tension free, deep dermal closure is completed with slowly resorbing monofilament suture (3-0 or 4-0 poliglecaprone 25) and skin with 5-0 or 6-0 nylon. Occasionally, the deep subcutaneous tissues require suspension to the orbitozygomatic periosteum to prevent scar widening or nasofacial groove flattening. This factor is important in wider flaps or where the donor site closure is tight. It is important to minimize undermining near the oral commissure and medial canthus because this will laterally distort these structures if closed under tension.

Modifications

The nasolabial flap may be harvested as a perforator based flap or island flap, which may be advantageous for nasal reconstruction.[3] By completely islanding the flap, a skin paddle can be tunneled subcutaneously to reconstruct nasal or cheek cutaneous defects not in continuity with the planned donor site. Monarca and colleagues[4] prospectively compared the use of traditional pedicled nasolabial flaps versus nasolabial island flaps in nasal ala reconstruction and demonstrated improved patient esthetic satisfaction scores and lower incidence of flap complications in the island group. When harvesting an island flap, it is important to carry the dissection in the supraperiosteal plane to include the facial artery and its perforators, because the subdermal plexus will be disrupted circumferentially. Failure to do so compromises vascular flow. Alternatively, a similar result can be obtained, particularly for intraoral reconstruction, by harvesting a standard thin pedicled nasolabial flap and carefully de-epithelializing the base. Although not a true island flap, it allows for subcutaneous tunneling into the oral cavity and complete donor site closure.[5]

Special considerations for recipient sites

Oral cavity reconstruction

For intraoral defects, notably floor of the mouth or buccal vestibular recipient sites, an inferiorly based flap is

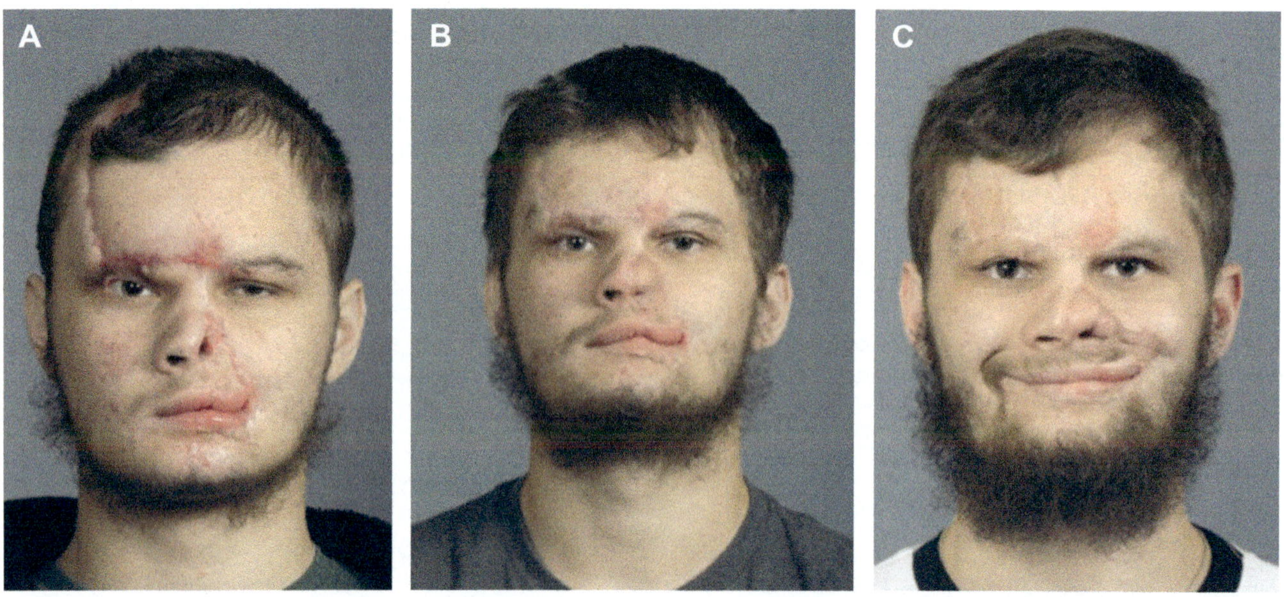

Fig. 1 (*A*) A 21-year-old man with left nasal ala soft tissue defect secondary to avulsive injury from motor vehicle accident. (*B*) Left nasal vestibular stenosis and obstruction noted after debridement and multiple local flaps, tissue expanders, and skin grafts for reconstruction. (*C*) The patient underwent a superiorly based left nasolabial flap with interpositional autogenous conchal cartilage graft to reconstruct his nasal ala. Division and inset was completed in the office under local anesthesia at 3 weeks postoperatively. Three-month postoperative photograph demonstrating left nasal patency with complete relief of his airflow obstruction.

preferred. The base should be of adequate width to capture subdermal blood supply, but not more than 2.5 cm, because excessive width will limit its arc of rotation into the oral cavity. The inferior limit of the flap should not extend past the oral commissure, because this will not improve reach and may cause lip and oral modiolus distortion when the donor site is closed. The flap must be passed through a transmucosal tunnel into the oral cavity. After elevation of the nasolabial flap, blunt dissection through the base of the donor site is completed with a hemostat toward the oral cavity. A counterincision can be made on the oral side through mucosa to connect the tunnel to the recipient site, and the flap is passed through with a traction suture or Allis clamp. Tension-free passage through a wide tunnel ensures that the flap does not become strangulated as postoperative edema worsens. In applications to the floor of mouth or palate, especially when the flap must cross the alveolus, a 2-stage approach is preferred. After adequate undermining and inset, the superior three-quarters of the donor site is closed, and the base of the flap is dressed with petrolatum gauze. Oftentimes, bilateral flaps are required for midline defects. In nonradiated patients, a latency period of at least 3 weeks is required before pedicle division. In patients with compromised vascular supply to the skin (radiation, diabetes, scleroderma), a longer interval may be necessary.

When the flap is ready to be divided, a 2-0 silk ligature is passed around the base and tightened to restrict blood flow. If capillary refill to the distal portion of the flap is intact, division may proceed. The base of the flap is divided with a scalpel while using a hemostat under it to protect the surrounding tissues. The donor site closure is completed and the final edge of the flap is inset to the medial portion of the recipient site.

Single-stage reconstruction is possible for smaller and well-lateralized defects of the oral cavity (buccal mucosa, labial vestibule). De-epithelializing the base of the flap before

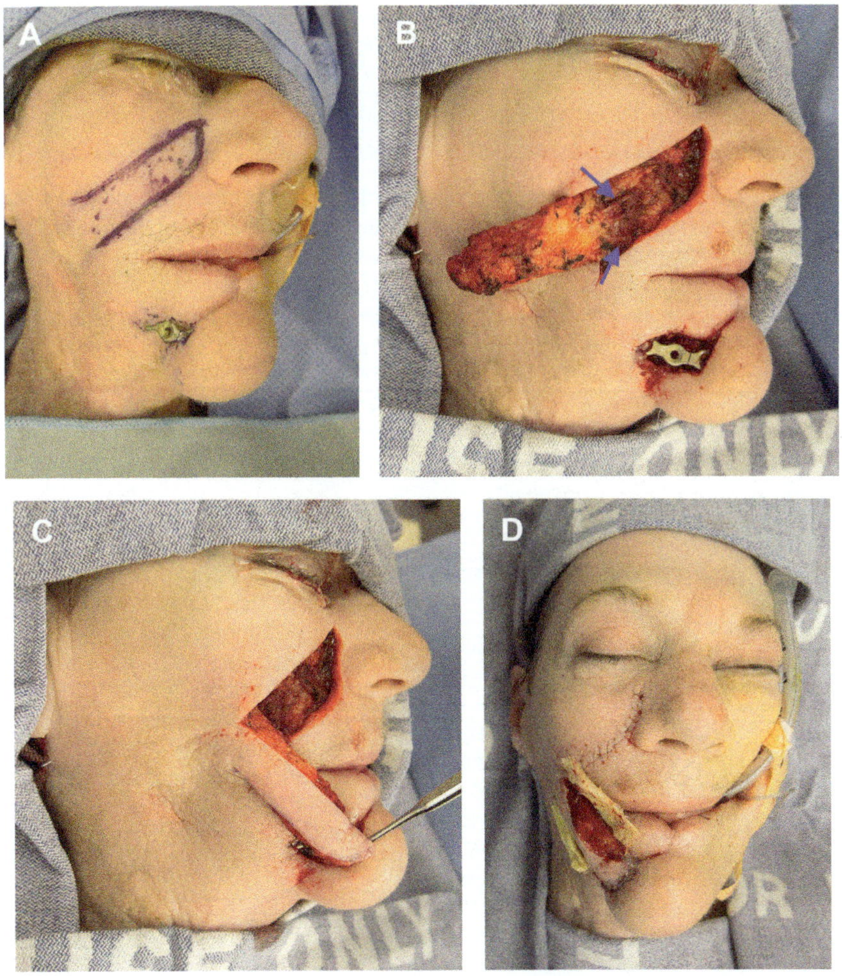

Fig. 2 (*A*) A 62-year-old woman with a history of multiple oral squamous cell carcinomas treated with surgery, radiotherapy, and chemotherapy. She now presents with exposure of her right mandibular reconstruction plate over a fibula free flap and vessel depleted neck. An inferiorly based nasolabial flap was designed to cover the exposed bone and mandibular plate using a 2-stage approach. Note the base of the flap is situated just above the level of the oral commissure. Superiorly, it is important to not encroach on the medial canthal region. (*B*) Harvest of a random pattern nasolabial flap and preparation and undermining of the recipient site. Bidigital palpation is helpful during harvest to maintain a uniform thickness. Small perforators were identified (*arrows*) and preserved during this dissection, but this is not a necessary step. (*C*) Adequate lateral undermining of the skin flap was required to reach the recipient site without difficulty. The flap can be extended slightly more inferiorly to improve reach if needed. (*D*) Inset of the flap in a tension-free manner and closure of the majority of the donor site. The exposed nonskin surfaces were dressed with petrolatum gauze for 4 weeks before pedicle division.

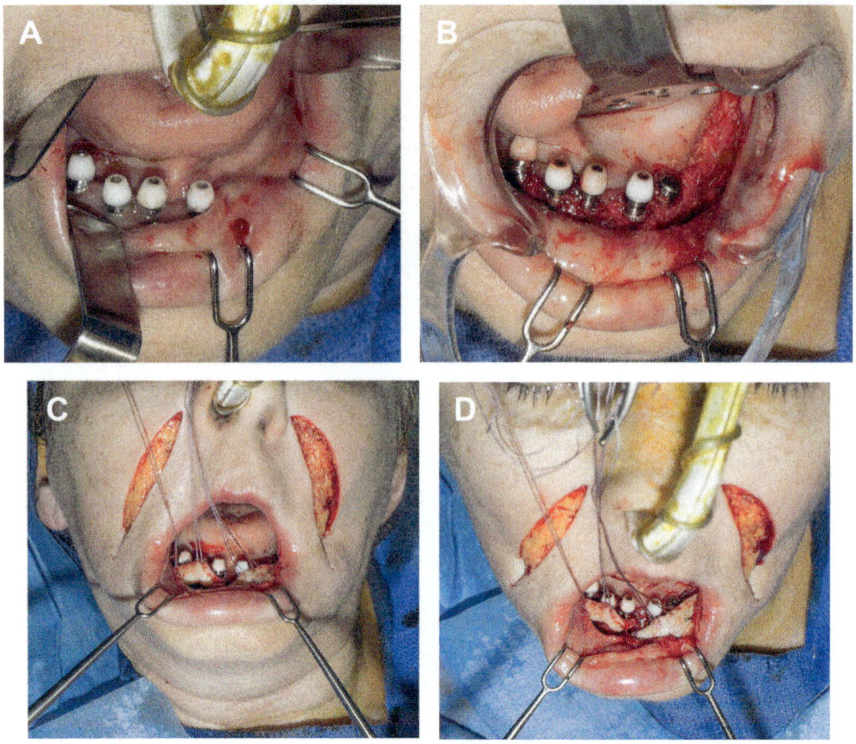

Fig. 3 (*A*) A 71-year-old woman with a history of scleroderma and multiple oral carcinoma in situ and floor of mouth squamous cell carcinoma status post excisions and local tissue rearrangement resulting in obliteration of her anterior mandibular vestibule and difficulty wearing her implant supported prosthesis. (*B*) Release of contracture between the labial mucosa and floor of mouth exposing the previously buried left mandibular dental implant. (*C*) Harvest and intraoral tunneling of bilateral inferiorly based random pattern nasolabial flaps. It is important to avoid the temptation to back cut the base of the flap to increase arc of rotation, because this maneuver will result in venous congestion of the flap. Careful undermining while maintaining the subdermal plexus allows each flap to reach just past the midline of the anterior mandibular vestibule. (*D*) Preliminary tension-free inset to complete the flap vestibuloplasty. Note that the apices of each flap overlap and cross the midline in a z-plasty fashion. This strategy decreases the likelihood of linear scar contraction and notching across the lip. The base of each flap was de-epithelialized for the length of the transbuccal tunnel and final inset and donor site closure completed in the standard fashion as described.

tunneling allows for complete skin closure over the donor site and inset.

Nasal ala reconstruction

The nasolabial flap is well-suited for nasal ala defects given its anatomic proximity and skin thickness and color match. As previously, the use of a nasolabial island flap for large nasal defects can be preferable, particularly if thick tissue is required. The benefit of superiorly pedicled thin nasolabial flaps for this application is the ability to sandwich a cartilage graft between a folded flap. By establishing the nasal framework with rib or ear cartilage, a thinned nasolabial flap can be folded over it and sutured to the remnant nasal mucosa, thereby vascularizing the cartilage and creating a function nasal vestibule.[6] As in oral cavity defects, this may be carried out as a single-stage or 2-stage operation, with the latter requiring a minimum period of 3 weeks before pedicle division.

Complications

The most dreaded complication of the nasolabial flap is vascular compromise and flap failure. Following the principles of skin flap physiology and proper preoperative evaluation mitigate this risk substantially. Avoiding a long narrow flap or excessively thinned flap is important in maintaining distal perfusion. Patients with microvasculopathy, such as those with uncontrolled diabetes mellitus, are at higher risk of flap ischemia or venous congestion.

Although the donor site falls within a natural facial crease, scarring can be problematic. Older patients with thinner skin and loss of elastin tolerate this donor site quite well with minimal long-term stigmata of flap harvest. Younger patients with minimal skin creases, thick and oily skin, or those with increased pigmentations may suffer from unfavorable facial scarring or asymmetry.

Cases

Cases 1 through 5 are presented in Figs. 1–5.

Disclosure

The authors have nothing to disclose.

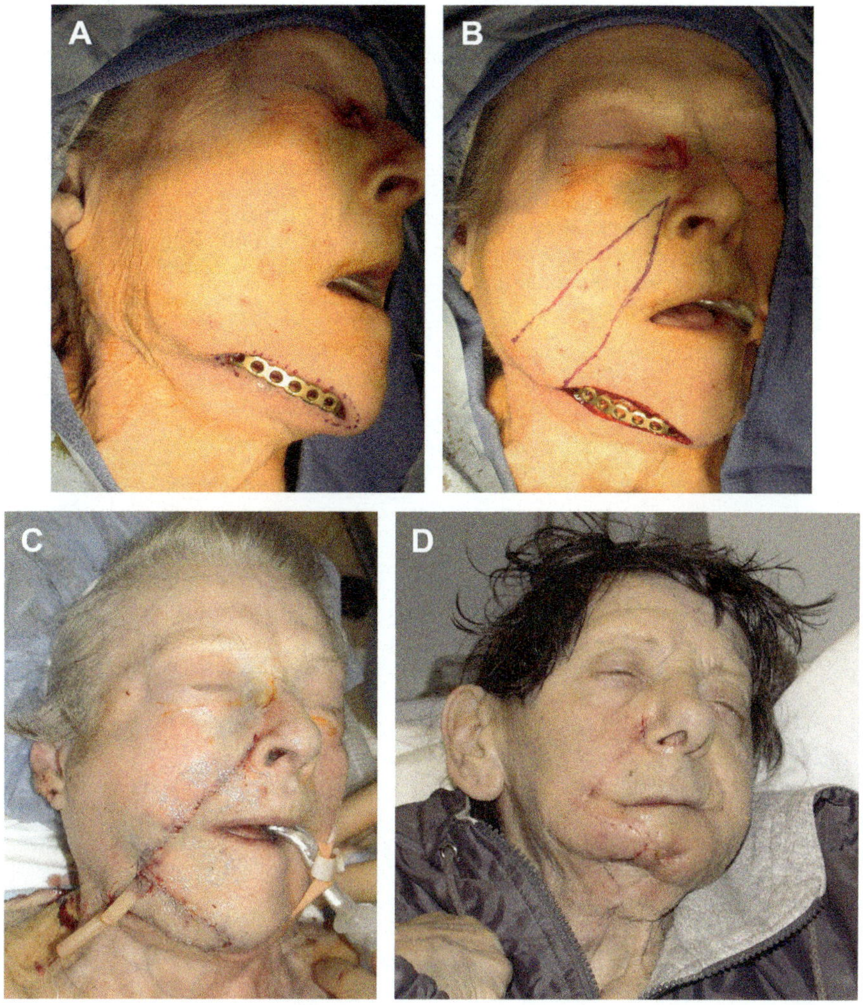

Fig. 4 (*A*) A 78-year-old man with a 6-cm exposure of a right mandibular reconstruction plate. (*B*) The wound has been debrided and margins sharply delineated. A large inferiorly based random pattern nasolabial transposition flap has been designed to provide vascularized soft tissue coverage of the wound. Note that the base of the flap required incision and dissection well below the oral commissure to allow for transposition in a single-stage approach. (*C*) The flap has been elevated in the subcutaneous plane and inset without tension to the inferior mandibular wound. The donor site was closed easily with lateral skin flap undermining. Penrose drains were placed to prevent hematoma formation, but are not always necessary. (*D*) Three-week postoperative follow-up photograph demonstrating excellent wound coverage, color match, and thickness match. Notice there is some distortion of the oral commissure, because the flap required extension below this level. (*Courtesy of* Eric J. Dierks MD, DMD, FACS, FRCS, FACD, Portland, OR.)

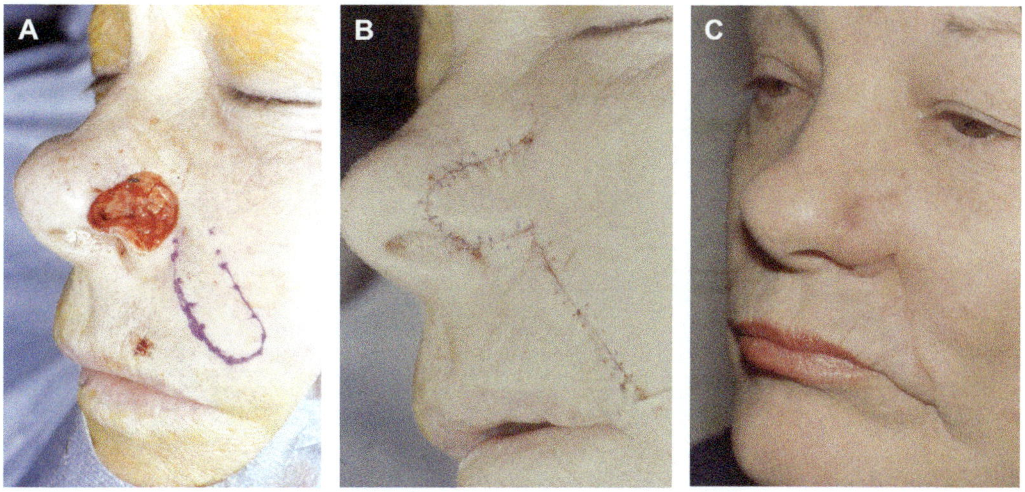

Fig. 5 (*A*) A 59-year-old woman status post Moh's micrographic excision of a left nasal alar squamous cell carcinoma. A superiorly based random pattern nasolabial transposition flap was designed to reconstruct the defect. It is important to not underestimate the length to allow for adequate arc of rotation and tension-free closure. The distal portion of the flap was harvested to match the thickness of the nasal defect. (*B*) Transposition of the flap and inset, as well as donor site closure. (*C*) Postoperative appearance with mild residual lymphedema and obliteration of the nasolabial crease at the base of the flap. (*Courtesy of* Eric J. Dierks MD, DMD, FACS, FRCS, FACD, Portland, OR.)

References

1. Zufferey JA. Is the malaris muscle the anti-aging missing link of the midface? Eur J Plast Surg 2013;36(6):345–52.
2. Memarzadeh K, Sheikh R, Blohmé J, et al. Perfusion and oxygenation of random advancement skin flaps depend more on the length and thickness of the flap than on the width to length ratio. Eplasty 2016;16:e12.
3. Horta R, Teixeira S, Nascimento R, et al. The freestyle facial artery perforator flap for reconstruction of simultaneous periorbital and cheek defects. J Craniofac Surg 2016;27(5):e473–4.
4. Monarca C, Rizzo MI, Palmieri A, et al. Comparative analysis between nasolabial and island pedicle flaps in the ala nose reconstruction. Prospective study. In Vivo 2012;26(1):93–8.
5. Ducic Y, Burye M. Nasolabial flap reconstruction of oral cavity defects: a report of 18 cases. J Oral Maxillofac Surg 2000;58(10):1104–8 [discussion 8–9].
6. Jovanović M, Colić M, Rasulić L, et al. Reconstruction of the alae nasi by folded nasolabial flap. Acta Chir Iugosl 2007;54(2):29–32 [in Serbian].

Cervicofacial Flap

Al Haitham Al Shetawi, MD, DMD

KEYWORDS

• Cheek reconstruction • Cervicofacial flap • Cervicopectoral flap

KEY POINTS

- The cervicofacial flap is a random pattern flap.
- The flap can be anteriorly or posteriorly based.
- The cervicofacial flap is an excellent option for medium- and large-sized cutaneous cheek defects.
- The cervicopectoral flap can be used in very large cheek defects.

Introduction: nature of the problem

There are numerous reconstructive options for cheek defects, such as primary closure, skin grafting, healing by secondary intention, and local, regional, or free flaps. The cervicofacial flap is the mainstay of reconstruction for medium- and large-sized cheek defects. It provides a large surface area with excellent color and texture match. A properly designed and elevated cervicofacial flap is an excellent and reliable choice to reconstruct cutaneous cheek defects.

Surgical technique

Preoperative planning

The choice of flap depends on intrinsic wound characteristics, such as size, depth, and anatomic location, and extrinsic factors, such as adjacent anatomic structures and patient's condition. The surgeon's creativity plays an essential role in flap selection. In general, cheek defects are preferably reconstructed with tissue from adjacent units, such as the neck, submental area, or chest. The cervicofacial flap is an excellent choice for medium to large cheek defects.

Preparation and patient positioning

The patient is placed in the supine position. The head is rotated toward the contralateral side, and the neck is extended. The ipsilateral face and neck are prepared and draped in the sterile technique. It is important to have the entire ipsilateral face in the field to monitor any twitching during flap elevation. The eyes should be protected with an occlusive dressing or shield. The chest is included in the field if the plan is to use a cervicopectoral flap. General anesthesia is usually used for this flap; however, local anesthesia and sedation can be used. The use of paralytic agents during general anesthesia is not contraindicated when needed.

Surgical approach

- The resection is carried out in the standard oncologic technique. For an anteriorly based flap, the flap is marked from the lateral border of the defect, extended lateral to a preauricular crease, and carried inferiorly around the earlobe and then to a cervical crease (Figs. 1A and 2A).
- The incision is made through the skin and subcutaneous fat along the markings (Figs. 1B and 2B).
- The flap is elevated in a plane superficial to the superficial musculoaponeurotic system in the face and parotid region and deep to the platysma in the neck (Figs. 1C and 2C). When the anterior margin of the parotid gland is reached, care should be taken to avoid injury to the facial nerve branches. In the cervical region, care should be taken to avoid injury to the greater auricular nerve.
- The flap is advanced to assess the reach. Flap elevation is stopped when adequate tension-free closure can be achieved. A wedge excision medial to the defect is performed to avoid forming a dog-ear deformity (Figs. 1D and 2D).
- The wound is closed in layers. A closed or an open system drain is placed to prevent seroma or hematoma formation (Figs. 1E and 2E). The drain is usually removed on the first postoperative day.
- Outcome is shown at 3 months' follow-up (Figs. 1F and 2F).

For very large defects, a cervicopectoral flap can be used (Fig. 3A, B).

- The incision is extended to the chest (Fig. 3C).
- The flap is elevated in the subplatysmal plane in the neck and suprafascial plane in the chest. Care should be taken in the midline chest to prevent injury to the internal mammary perforators (Fig. 3D).
- The reach of the flap is assessed to ensure tension-free closure (Fig. 3E).

Division of Surgical Oncology, Department of Surgery, Vassar Brother Medical Center, Nuvance Health, Dyson Center for Cancer Care, 45 Reade Place, 3rd Floor, Poughkeepsie, NY 12603, USA
E-mail addresses: al-haitham.al-shetawi@nuvancehealth.org, aalsheta@health-quest.org

Atlas Oral Maxillofacial Surg Clin N Am 28 (2020) 13-15
1061-3315/20/© 2019 Elsevier Inc. All rights reserved.
https://doi.org/10.1016/j.cxom.2019.11.001

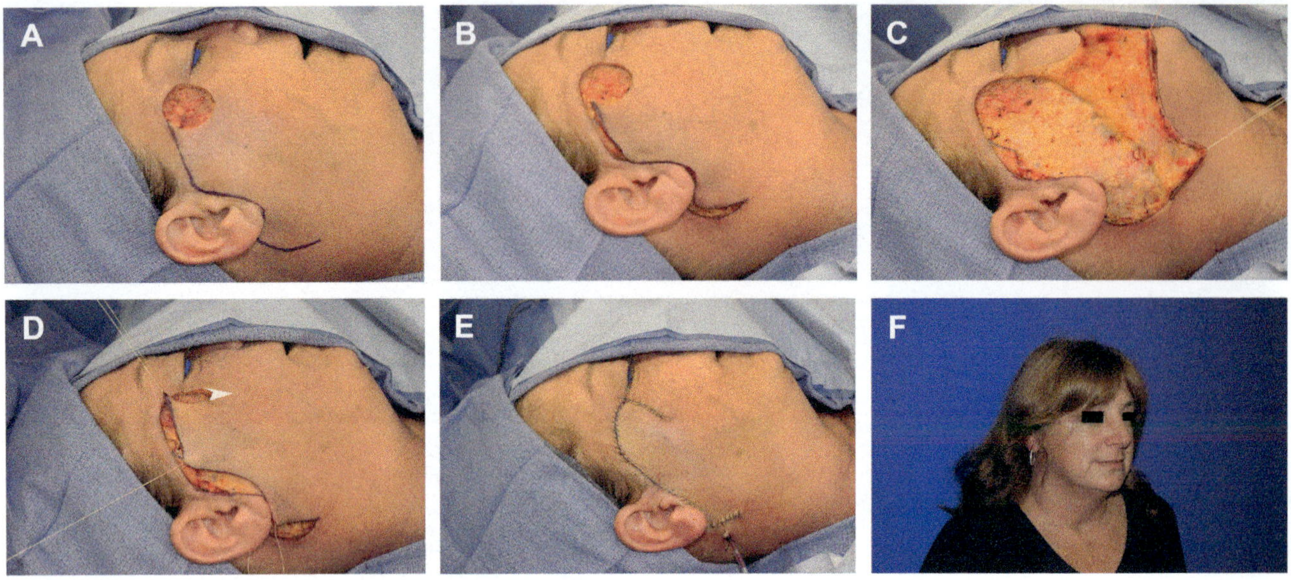

Fig. 1 Flap marking (*A*), incision (*B*), flap elevation (*C*), advancement and medial wedge excision (*D*), closure and drain placement (*E*), outcome (*F*).

- The flap is closed in layers over a suction drain (Fig. 3F).
- Outcome is shown at 3 months' follow-up (Fig. 3G).

Potential complications

The cervicofacial flap is a random pattern flap. To avoid distal flap necrosis, a wide base should be included in the flap design. An alternative method of reconstruction should be considered in a previously operated neck or radiated patients. In patients with composite cheek defect, this flap provides a limited tissue volume, and contour deformity can occur (see Fig. 3G).

Pearls and pitfalls

The flap elevation is easier to start at the defect. In the cervical region, care should be taken to avoid injury to the greater auricular nerve branches. When possible, incisions should be placed within facial creases and grooves (eg, the subciliary line, the nasofacial groove, and the preauricular crease).

Immediate postoperative care

Pressure dressing should be avoided to minimize distal flap necrosis. An open or closed suction drain is usually used to prevent seroma or hematoma accumulation.

Clinical results in the literature

The first form of cheek flap was introduced by Esser in 1918.[1] Several modifications to the flap were seen over the years until Juri and Juri[2] described the advancement rotational cervicofacial flap. The cheek is the largest unit in the face. It is bound superiorly by the infraorbital rim and the zygomatic arch, medially by the nasofacial junction, nasolabial fold, and

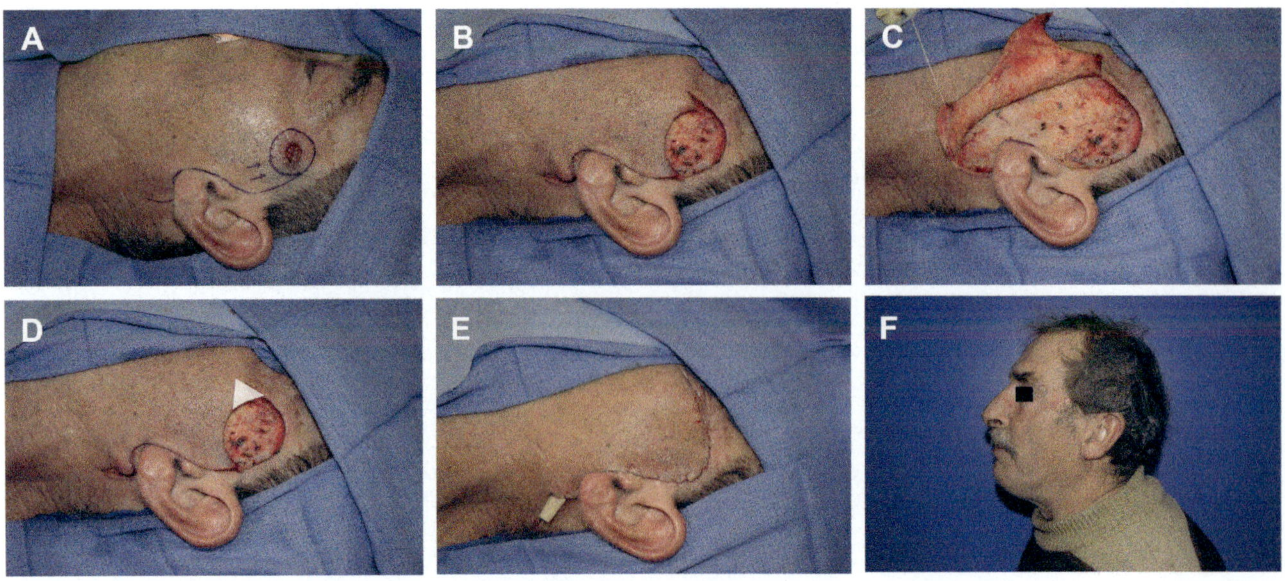

Fig. 2 Flap marking (*A*), incision (*B*), flap elevation (*C*), advancement and medial wedge excision (*D*), closure and drain placement (*E*), outcome (*F*).

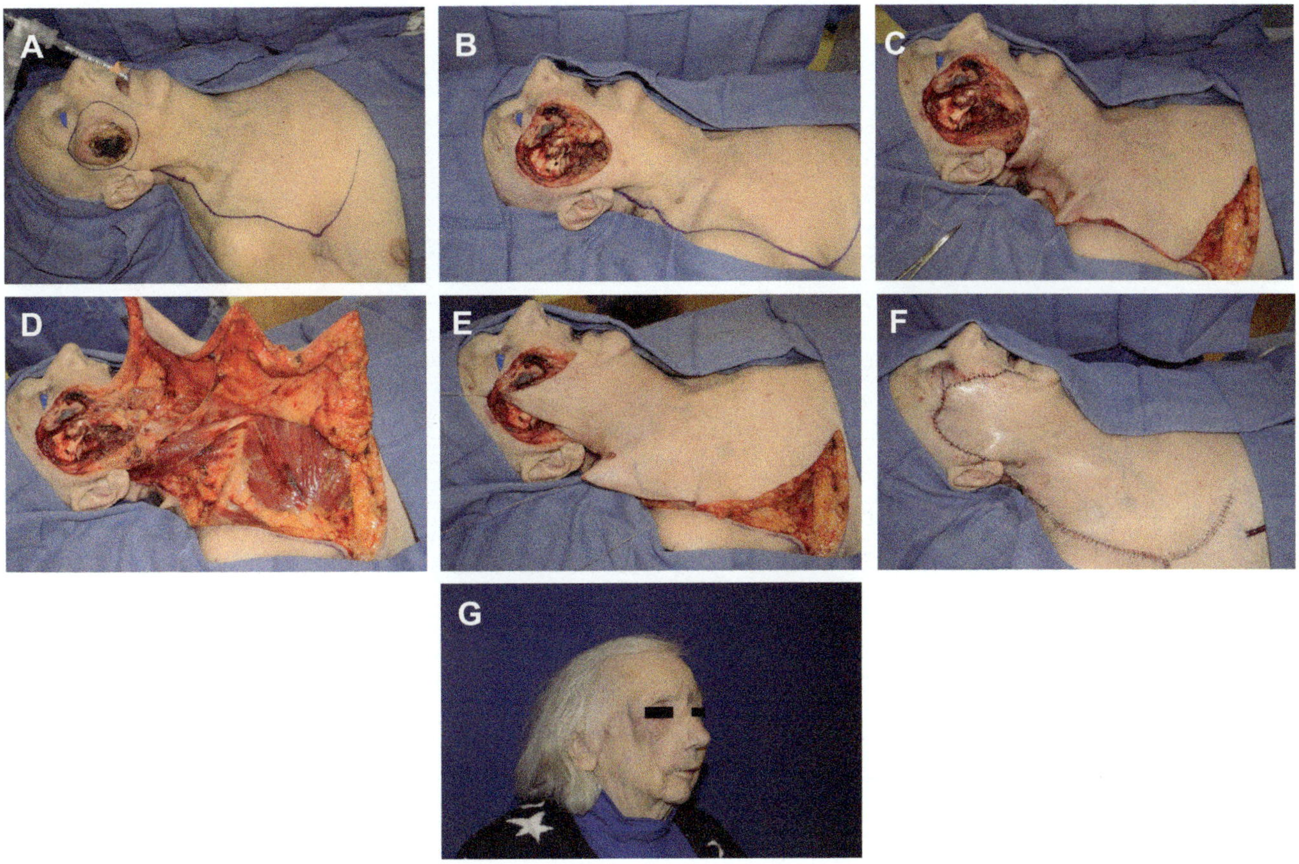

Fig. 3 Large cheek tumor (*A*), flap marking (*B*), incision (*C*), flap elevation (*D*), advancement (*E*), closure and drain placement (*F*), outcome (*G*).

labiomandibular crease, inferiorly by the border of the mandible, and laterally by the preauricular crease.[3] Numerous options are available for reconstruction, such as primary closure, skin graft, healing by secondary intention, and local, regional, and free flaps.[4] The cervicofacial flap is the mainstay of reconstruction for medium- and large-sized cheek defects.[5] This flap can be an anteriorly based flap supplied by the facial and submental arteries or a posteriorly based flap supplied by the superficial temporal artery and preauricular vessels in the face[6] With good planning and flap elevation, this flap provides excellent skin color, thickness, and texture match in cheek reconstruction.[7]

Summary

A properly designed and elevated cervicofacial flap is an excellent and reliable choice to reconstruct medium- and large-sized cutaneous cheek defects.

Disclosure

The author has nothing to disclose.

References

1. Esser JFS. Die Rotation der Wange und allgemeine Bemerkungen bei chirurgischer Gesichtsplastik. Leipzig, Vogel; 1918.
2. Juri J, Juri C. Advancement and rotation of a large cervicofacial flap for cheek repairs. Plast Reconstr Surg 1979;64(5):692–6.
3. Dobratz EJ, Hilger PA. Cheek defects. Facial Plast Surg Clin North Am 2009;17(3):455–67.
4. Menick FJ. Reconstruction of the cheek. Plast Reconstr Surg 2001; 108(2):496–505.
5. Liu FY, Xu ZF, Li P, et al. The versatile application of cervicofacial and cervicothoracic rotation flaps in head and neck surgery. World J Surg Oncol 2011;9:135.
6. Mureau MA, Hofer SO. Maximizing results in reconstruction of cheek defects. Clin Plast Surg 2009;36(3):461–76.
7. Al Shetawi AH, Quimby A, Fernandes R. The cervicofacial flap in cheek reconstruction: a guide for flap design. J Oral Maxillofac Surg 2017;75(12):2708.e1-6.

Further readings

Fernandes R. Local and regional flaps in head & neck reconstruction: a practical approach. Ames (IA): Wiley Blackwell; 2015. p. 92–102. Chapter 13: Cervicofacial advancement flap.

Rhomboid Flap

Heidi H. Hon, MD [a,b],
Srinivasa Rama Chandra, MD, BDS, FDSRCS(Eng), FIBCSOMS (Onc- Recon) [a,b,*]

KEYWORDS

• Rhomboid flap • Rhombic flap • Transposition flap • Limberg flap • Rotational flap • Dufourmentel flap • Local pedicle flap • Local facial flaps

KEY POINTS

- The rhomboid flap is a workhorse flap for reconstruction of facial and head and neck defects based on the transposition flap design.
- The rhomboid excision (60° and 120° angles) should parallel the skin tension line in the longitudinal axis.
- Disadvantages of this transposition flap are tension, incision in healthy native tissue leading to secondary scar, and the potential for excess "dog-ear" tissue.
- Multiple modifications have been described to reduce the side effects as mentioned above, to decrease pivotal restraint and minimize tension to the tip of the flap.

Introduction

Facial cutaneous defects of noncritical sizes are reconstructed with local flaps, which are advanced, rotated, or transposed into the area. Among these local flaps, the rhomboid flap is a geometrically random pattern—designed simple transposition flap. It follows the principles of flap design, retaining its vascularity from the connected limb of adequate width, with its tissue composition similar to the excised region.

Historical perspective

Alexander A. Limberg, a maxillofacial surgeon from Russia, introduced this original concept of transposing a rhomboid-shaped flap 120° for closure of a similarly shaped defect in 1946.[1–6] As a result, this rhomboid flap is also described as the Limberg flap. The original Russian monograph, *Mathematical principles of local plastic procedures on the surface of the human body*, was subsequently published in 1966 in English as a "Design of local flaps" chapter for a plastic surgery textbook.[1–6] Since that time, multiple modifications to his flap design have been proposed. In 1966, a modified technique was described by Claude Dufourmentel, whereby angles between 60 and 90° were designed for the local tissue transfer. Therefore, less healthy tissue was disturbed for the transposition with a wider pedicle width of the local flap. About a decade later, in 1978, Richard Webster described the 30° flap, whereby the distal flap is angulated only 30°, which helped with tip ischemia. However, closure of the defect base required an M-plasty, which helped minimize tension to the flap. In 1987, another modification surfaced known as the Quaba/Sommerlad flap, which was designed to close circular defects.[7] The design of the transposed flap was smaller than that of the defect, and the defect was not converted to a geometric rhomboid-shaped defect.

It is interesting to note the origin and evolution of the Greek word *rhombos* (Latin *rhombus*) and the derivative words rhomboid and rhombic. The original term *rhombos* predates the Euclidian era and was the name used in ancient Greece for the spinning top toy.[1–6] The familiar shape of a spinning toy is a symmetric quadrilateral (usually not a parallelogram) with equal adjacent sides and having at least 2 of its 4 angles being equal. Later on, this definition was slightly changed by Euclidian geometry to denote the well-known shape of a parallelogram with 4 equal sides, opposite equal acute angles, and opposite equal obtuse angles (excluding the square). It therefore becomes obvious that the use of the term rhomboid (or rhombic) to describe the flap of Limberg is based on the Euclidian definition of the rhombus shape and not the one corresponding to the shape of the spinning top toy. It is also significant to clarify that the terms rhomboid (having shape/characteristics like that of a rhombus) and rhombic (having the shape/characteristics of a rhombus) are closely related, with the term rhombic being a slightly more precise descriptor of the Limberg flap (Fig. 1).

Indications and contraindications

Small to medium defects that are too large for primary closure are very amenable to reconstruction with transposition flaps. For instance, anatomic subunits, including the forehead,

[a] Division of Plastic and Reconstruction Surgery, Department of Surgery, University of Nebraska Medical Center, 984125, Specialist surgery pavilion - Room 2018, Nebraska Medicine, Omaha, NE 68198-4125, USA
[b] Division of OMFS—Head and Neck Surgery, Head and Neck Oncology and Microvascular Reconstructive Surgery, Department of Surgery, University of Nebraska Medical Center, Fred & Pamela Buffett Cancer Center, Omaha, NE, USA
* Corresponding author.
E-mail address: sriniRchandra4@gmail.com

Atlas Oral Maxillofacial Surg Clin N Am 28 (2020) 17-22
1061-3315/20/© 2019 Elsevier Inc. All rights reserved.
https://doi.org/10.1016/j.cxom.2019.11.005

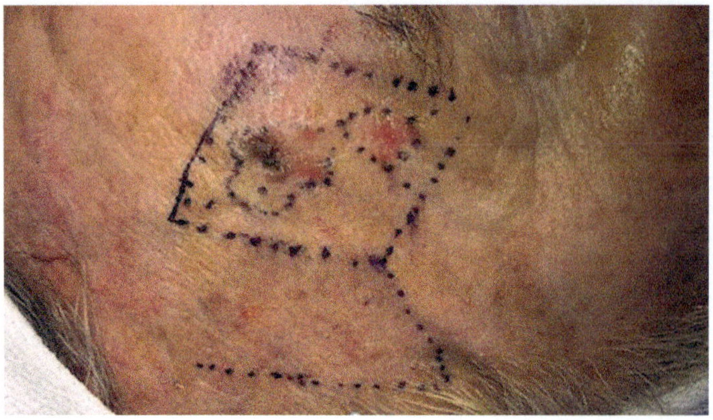

Fig. 1 Rhomboid or Limberg flap design showing 2 symmetric and opposing equal angles.

malar, temple, and the inferior part of the chin and lip, are ideal locations for vector transposition using the rhomboid flap in the resting skin tension lines. Inadequate margin resection is an absolute contraindication to any reconstructive option until margins are negative from the oncologic standpoint. Relative contraindications include patient factors, such as anti-coagulation, radiation history, impaired vascularity, previous local tissue rearrangement, and immunosuppressive pharmacologic considerations.

Surgical considerations

Rhomboid flaps are used in various anatomic regions of the entire body, making it an extremely versatile flap given its ability to reconstruct defects with similar tissue of texture and color. It has been demonstrated to be very useful in pilonidal cyst defects. However, it is still most commonly used in the face, head, and neck regions. For the maxillofacial surgeon, the rhomboid flap has great use in the temporal, periocular regions, nasal bridge, cheek/malar areas, chin, and neck regions. Pathologic condition, adequate margin resection, diameter of the lesion, scar orientation, area of maximal tension upon closure, skin laxity, and future reconstructive options (if necessary) are important considerations in any local flap reconstruction. The reconstructive ladder begins from secondary intention to free tissue transfer with the role of local or pedicled flaps chosen as an option for small to medium defects, which are aesthetically amenable to closure. Fillers, chemotherapeutic medications, lasers, scar modifiers like dermabrasion, and microneedling are additional adjunctive reconstructive aids to correct pin-cushioning or dog-ear deformities.

Anesthetic considerations

Vital considerations for an anesthetic evaluation include the patient's medical history, medication allergies, family history, and compliance during the procedure. Most transposition flaps are amenable to local and regional anesthesia with or without sedation. General anesthesia is certainly a consideration for surgical execution in an anatomically complex defect, poor pain tolerance, and so forth.

Flap design

The essence of the donor site closure and reconstruction should minimize distortion of adjacent structures. Previous scars, muscle, and ligament attachments, like the lateral canthus, for instance, must be accounted for. The relaxed skin tension lines and vectors are identified before flap design (Fig. 2). The line of the incision in adjacent normal donor skin is parallel to the relaxed skin tension lines, and the short-axis incision extension is placed within the lines of maximal extensibility (Fig. 3).[8] In the absence of obvious skin folds or creases, a pinch test of the skin would guide orientation. The base of the flap is the most important part of the flap design because it will maintain flap viability. The base of the pedicle should not be narrowed or undercut, and the flap design should account for anatomic subunits and tension lines to prevent stretching or tethering of the vasculature of flap.

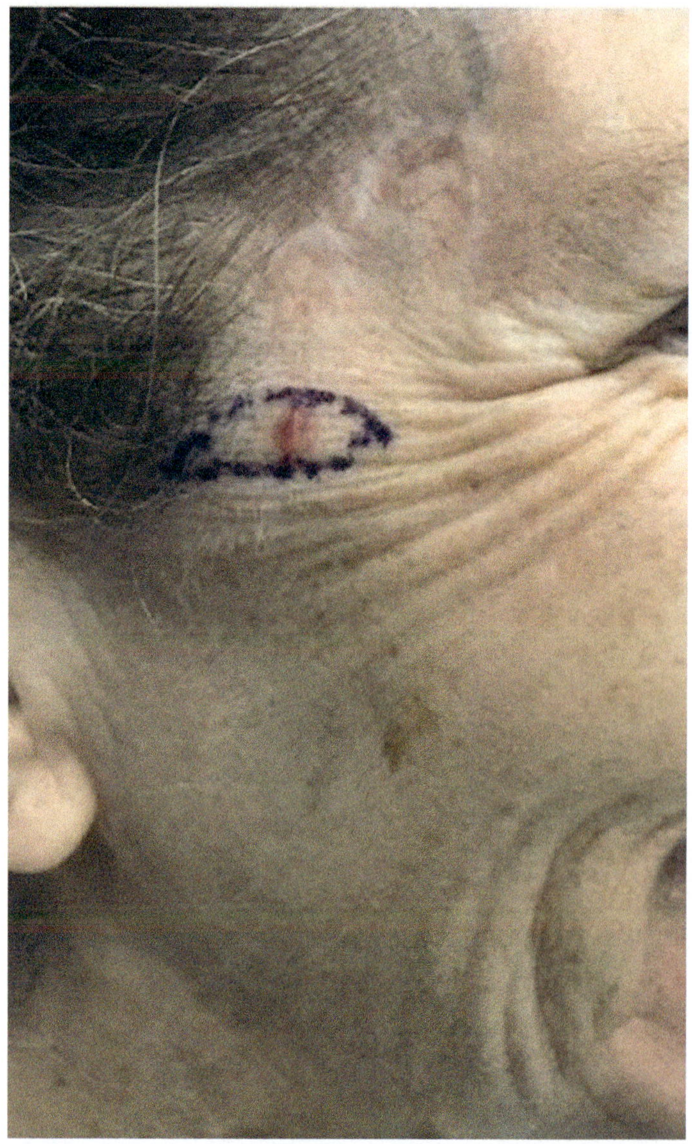

Fig. 2 The resting skin tension lines (RSTL) of the right facial region. The previous transposition flap is well healed, and the current lesion is well positioned in the RSTL.

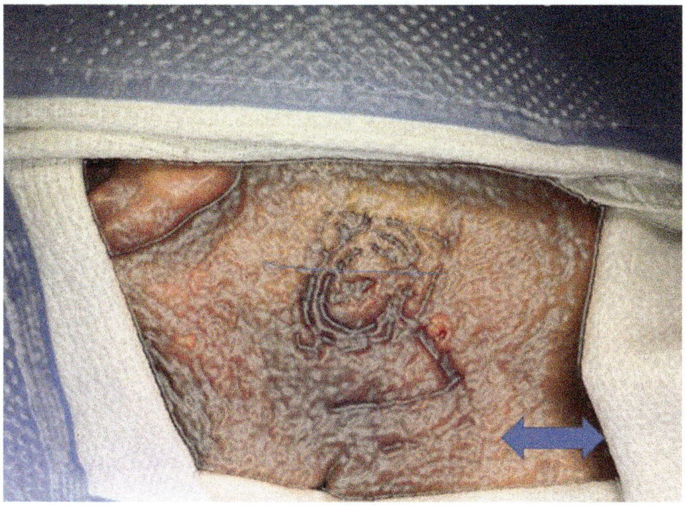

Fig. 3 The key to location of the vectors of pull. The line of the incision in adjacent normal donor skin is parallel to the RSTL (*thin curved line*), and the short-axis incision extension is in the lines of maximal extensibility (*thick double-ended arrow*).

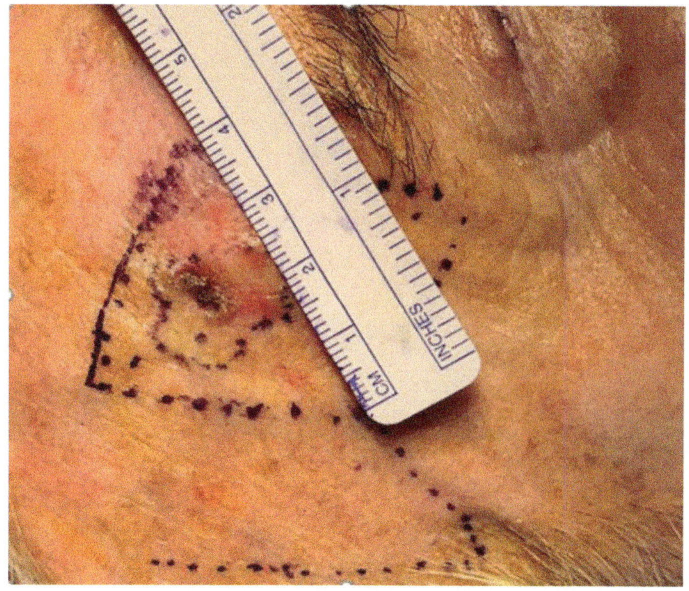

Fig. 5 The orientation of the 2 possible flaps is evaluated. Efforts are to minimize the distortion of the adjacent aesthetic subunit anatomy, such as the lateral canthus of the eye shown here.

Surgical technique

The defect is outlined as a geometric rhombus for the concept of flap design (Fig. 4). The axis between the two 60° angles of the rhombus serves as the "long axis." The "short axis" is the distance between the 2 obtuse 120° angles. Incisions are designed within resting skin tension lines when possible. The geometric rhombus with 2 opposing 60° angles and two opposing 120° angles is then outlined with 4 possibilities of flap design around this geometric rhombus. The orientation and the surrounding anatomic subunit consideration for tissue tension and scar placement should influence the decision on which possibility would be most appropriate (Fig. 5). The secondary defect and scar should lay with the least amount of tension on the donor site.

Bipolar electrocautery during flap harvest is recommended to ensure hemostasis and prevention of hematoma. The first incision of this design is the limb off the 120° angle short axis. The first incision should be of equal length to the sides of the geometric rhombus. The second limb of the incision is at 60° to the first limb and parallel to the side of the defect. Depth of the transposition flap should be equal to the depth of the defect to maintain continuity to achieve an optimal aesthetic outcome (Fig. 6). Adjacent tissue is elevated in a similar plane to assist with closure. The flap is rotated into the

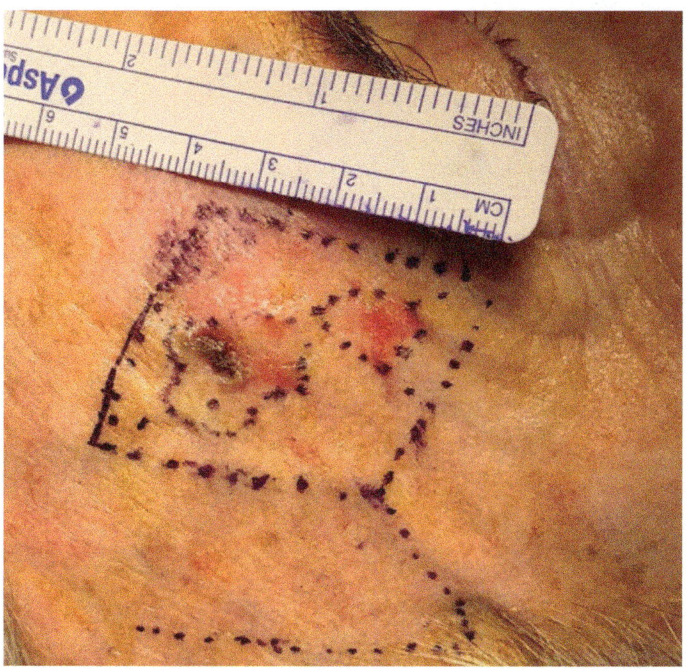

Fig. 4 Rhomboid or Limberg flap design showing 2 symmetric and opposing equal angles. Any cutaneous lesion can be geometrically planned into a rhomboid flap.

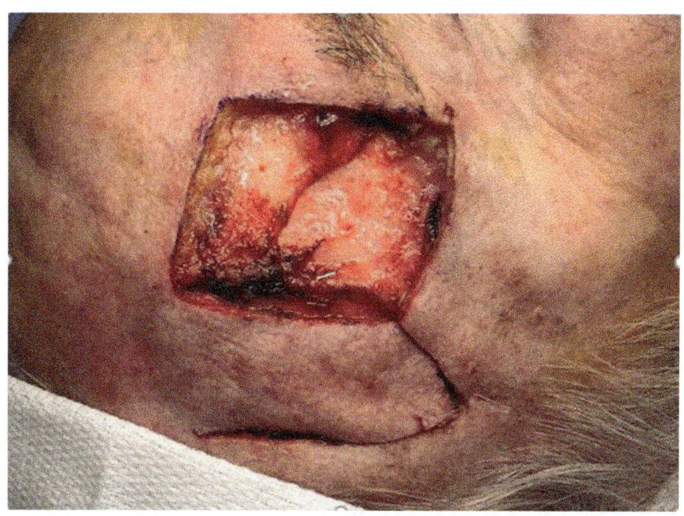

Fig. 6 The depth of the defect in the rhombus should equal the depth of excision in the normal tissue limb elevated for transposition.

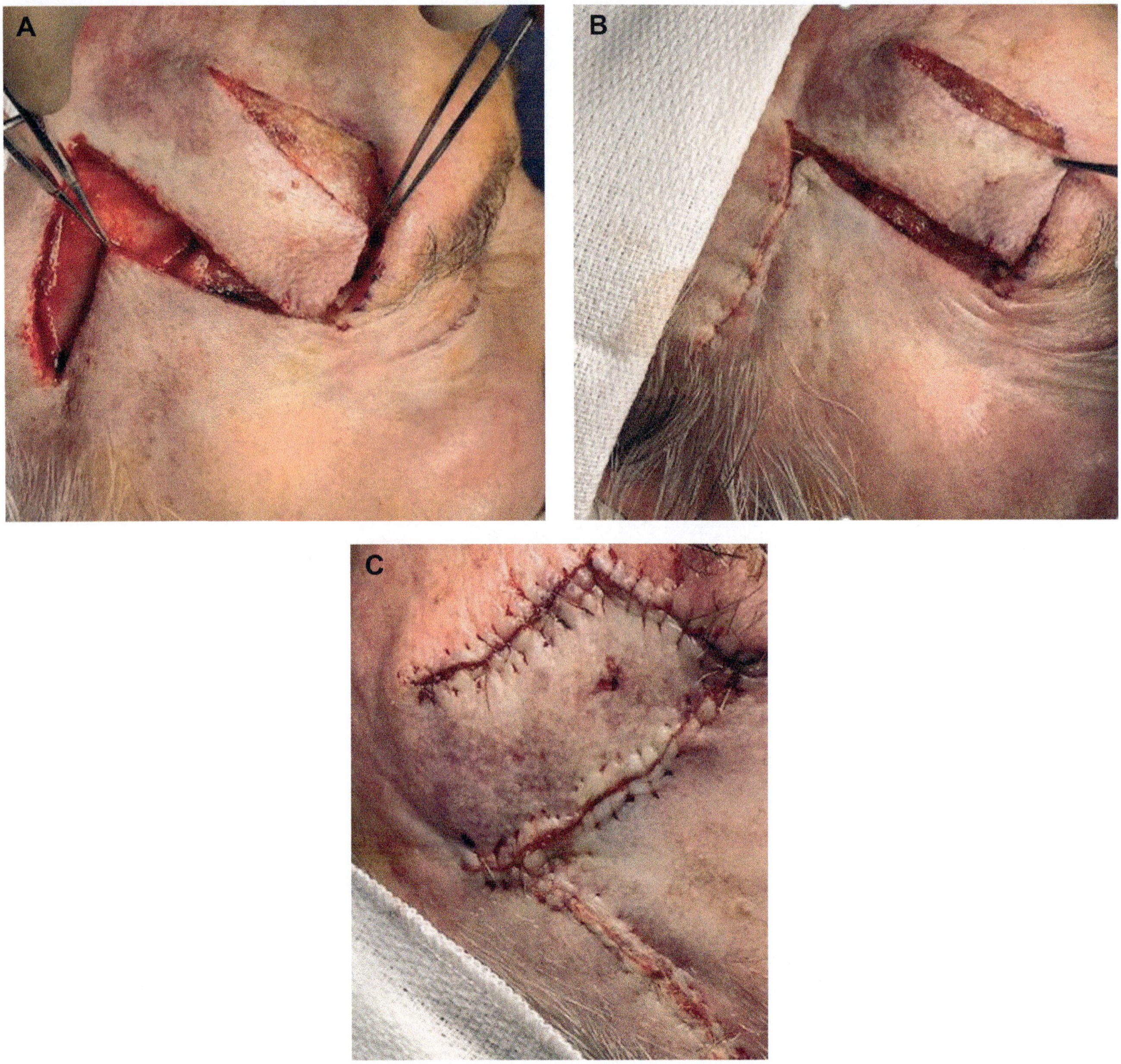

Fig. 7 (*A*) Depiction of transposition of the flap with evaluation of adjacent soft tissue distortion. Here the lateral cantus of the eye and the pliability of the flap are being evaluated. (*B*) Secondary defect is closed first. (*C*) Final closure with deep and skin closure.

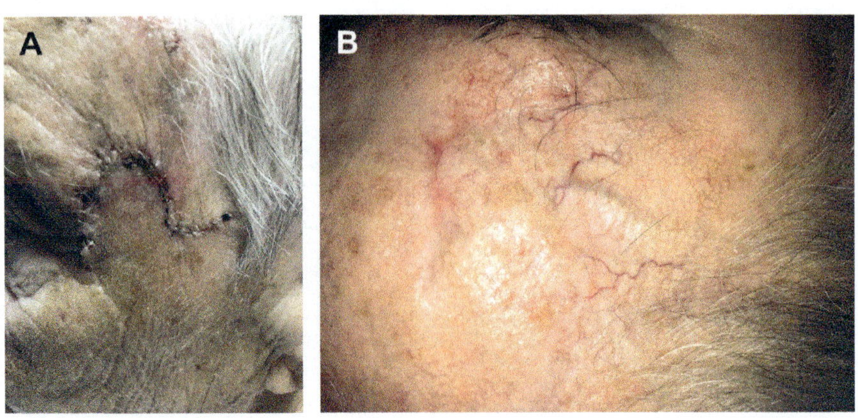

Fig. 8 (*A*) The final scar appears like a question mark (*?*), with the lower limb pointing laterally in the illustration. (*B*) Postoperative 12-week follow-up result of the rhomboid flap.

defect to assess for tension and distortion of adjacent structures (Fig. 7A). The donor site is closed first (Fig. 7B), and the flap is then inset with care not to strangulate the corners of the transposed limb (Fig. 7C). The skin sutures can be absorbable or nonabsorbable and placed in a simple interrupted or mattress pattern when necessary. The final scar appears in the shape of a "question mark" (Fig. 8A, B).

Pearls and pitfalls

What is pivotal restraint?

Any arc of rotation is limited (restrained) by the length of axis and tissue at the pivot point, which is called pivotal restraint. As a result, tension will be present at the tip of the flap during flap inset. Optimal undermining at the pivot areas without compromising vascular viability is essential. Larrabee and colleagues[8] concluded that the greatest amount of tension for the rhomboid flap is present at closure of the donor site; this must be taken into consideration when undermining adjacent tissue to assist with closure.

Dufourmentel modification

Dufourmentel flap modification of the rhomboid flap was proposed as a right-angle (90°) variation for a shorter arc of rotation than the classic Limberg proposal.[9,10] The reduced 90° angle can also be modified to even smaller angles between 60° and 90°. The dashed line represents the Dufourmentel design (Fig. 9). Advantages of this modification include decreasing pivotal restraint, resulting in less tension on the tip, and a wider pedicle width.

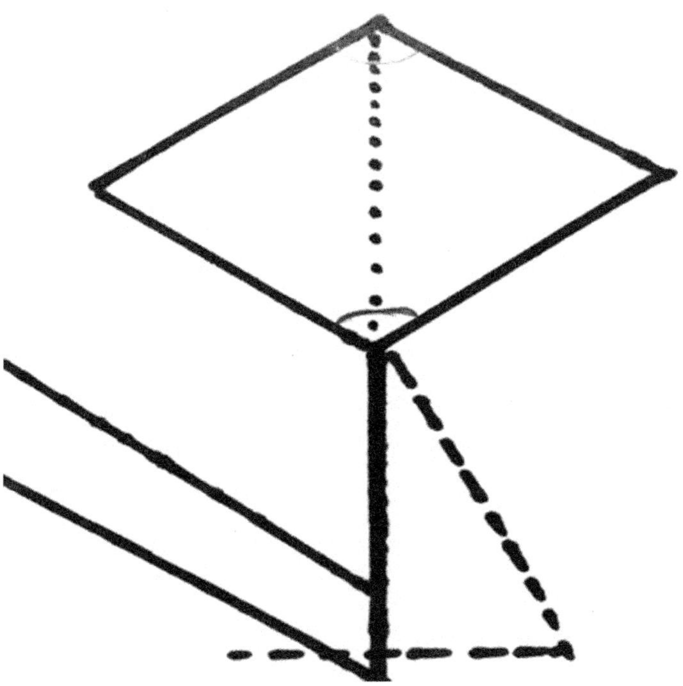

Fig. 9 Dufourmentel modification: Lengthening all sides and reduced angles closer to 30°, less than 60°. The dotted line is the incision, and the thick lines are the original parallels of rhomboid flap.

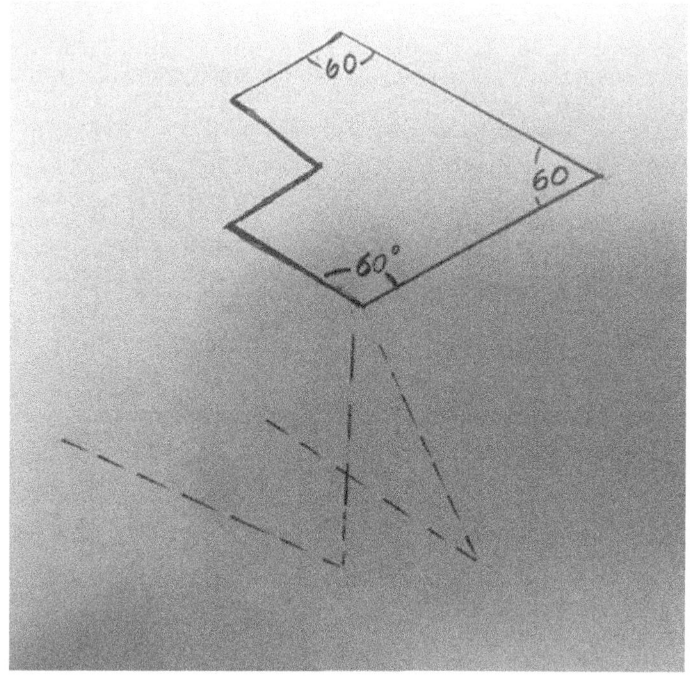

Fig. 10 Webster Modification: To reduce tension and aid closure of the 60° flap, Webster and colleagues,[11] in 1978, proposed a 30° flap tip angle combined with M-plasty. This M-plasty reduces the rotational deformity at the edges. As the flap tip reduces from 60° to 30°, the width of the flap is reduced (see Fig. 2). The dotted lines indicate the incision design options.

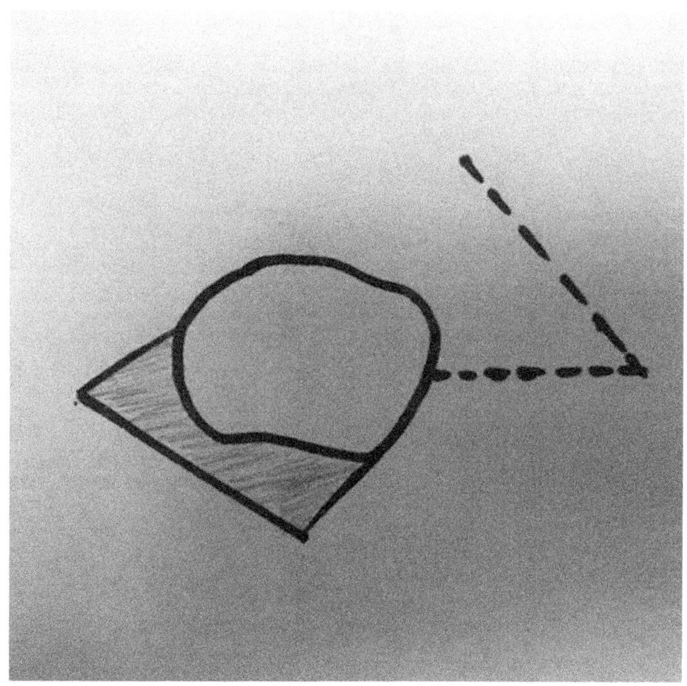

Fig. 11 Other modifications can be performed with defect edges removed in a geometric fashion to transpose a flap arm and reconstruct defects. The shaded areas are removed; the defect is converted to symmetric region, and the dotted lines are the planned incision.

Webster modification

To reduce tension and aid closure of the donor site, Webster and colleagues[11] proposed a 30° flap tip angle combined with M-plasty. This M-plasty reduces the rotational deformity at the edges. As the flap tip angle reduces from 60° to 30°, the base of the pedicle is increased (Fig. 10).

Other modifications can be performed with defect edges removed in a geometric fashion (Fig. 11). The shaded areas are removed; the defect is converted to symmetric region, and the dotted lines are the planned incision.

Acknowledgments

The corresponding author would like to express sincere thanks to Dr Prof Irkalis I. Pipinos, MD, FACS for his insight into the Greek translations and Euclid documents.

Disclosure

The authors have nothing to disclose.

References

1. Limberg AA. Mathematical principles of local plastic procedures the surface of the body. Leningrad (Russia): Medgis; 1946.
2. Limberg AA. Design of local flaps. In: Gibson T, editor. Modern trends in plastic surgery, vol. 2. London: Butterworth; 1966. p. 38–61.
3. Ardelt M, Settmacher U. Limberg flap is rhombic, not rhomboid. Plast Reconstr Surg 2016;137(2):494e–5e.
4. Limberg AA. The planning of local plastic operations on the body surface: theory and practice. Wolfe Lexington (MA): Collamore; 1984. p. 576. translated into English by S. A.
5. Pavlidis L, Spyropoulou GA. Limberg flap is rhombic, not rhomboid. Plast Reconstr Surg 2016;138(3):564e–5e.
6. Euclid's Elements of Geometry: The Greek text of J.L. Heiberg (1883–1885). Euclidis Elementa, edidit et Latine interpretatus est I.L. Heiberg, in aedibus B.G. Teubneri, 1883–1885 (Translation edited by Richard Fitzatrick). First Edition 2007 Revised and corrected - 2008; ISBN 978-0-6151-7984-1.
7. Quaba AA, Sommerlad BC. A square peg into a round hole: a modified rhomboid flap and its clinical applications. Br J Plast Surg 1987;40:163–70.
8. Larrabee WF Jr, Trachy R, Sutton D, et al. Rhomboid flap dynamics. Arch Otolaryngol 1981;107(12):755–7.
9. Dufourmentel C. La fermeture des pertes de substance cutanee limitees: le lambeau de rotation en L pour losange dit"LLL.". Ann Chir Plast 1962;7:61.
10. Dufourmentel C. An L-shaped flap for lozenge shaped defects: principle–technique–applications. Transact Third Int Congr Plast Surg. Amsterdam: Excerpta Medica; 1964. p. 772–3.
11. Webster RC, Davidson TM, Smith RC. The thirty-degree transposition flap. Laryngoscope 1978;88:85.

Paramedian Forehead Flap

Daniel Hammer, DDS*, Fayette Williams, DDS, MD, Roderick Kim, DDS, MD

KEYWORDS

• Nasal reconstruction • Head and neck reconstruction • Regional flap • Moh's excision • Skin cancer • Pedicled flap • Interpolated flap • Staged reconstruction

KEY POINTS

- The paramedian forehead flap is a reliable flap for reconstruction of extensive nasal defects.
- The flap can be completed in 1, 2, or 3 stages depending on the patient's defect, comorbidities, and patient desires.
- The flap has very low failure rates, with the most common complications being local infection and distal flap necrosis.
- The overall patient satisfaction with this flap is very high, with few patients needing multiple refinement procedures.

Introduction

Reconstruction of central facial defects is challenging and the efforts must establish precise outlines and positions to reestablish facial symmetry. Numerous etiologies for nasal skin defects (pathologic, traumatic, congenital, infectious, etc) must be taken into consideration for flap design. Reconstructive goals include restoration of nasal form and function (airflow), incorporating proper nasal dimension, volume, position, and contour. The reconstruction chosen must consider the patient's nasal deformity (size, depth, and subunits involved), available donor sites, patient's comorbidities, and the patient's desired outcome. For the reconstruction of full-thickness, large nasal defects, the interpolated, multilaminar paramedian forehead flap provides excellent results to restore patient's form and function.

Surgical technique

Preoperative planning

The most important factor regarding successful flap reconstruction is proper planning. This begins with the initial clinical examination with key points highlighted in Table 1.

Preparation and patient positioning

- Supine
- Oral intubation with Mastisol and Tegaderm on the upper lip to seal the oral cavity without distorting lip and cheek position
- A 20 to 30° reverse Trendelenburg to decrease venous pooling and blood loss
- Corneal shields with Lacrilube placed
- 10% Providine preparation

Surgical approach

For the purpose of this article, we assume that nasal lining and substructures are present with a defect not amenable to other local flap reconstruction options owing to the size of the defect and the patient's desired aesthetic outcomes. The patient elects for a paramedian forehead flap as the reconstructive option owing to its superior color, texture, size, versatility, low morbidity, and aesthetic result. However, the surgeon must determine how many stages are needed for the patient's best functional and aesthetic outcome. Table 2 summarizes the indications for each type of staging and what each stage entails.

Surgical procedure (2-stage paramedian forehead flap)

Stage I

- Step 1: Marking patient
  - Involved nasal subunits identified and uninvolved normal tissue in affected convex subunits (tip and ala) are included for planned excision to avoid pin cushion defect and allow for improved scar camouflage (Fig. 1A, B)
  - Central nasal defects can be reconstructed with left- or right-based flap.
  - Lateral nasal defects should be reconstructed with ipsilateral flap, when possible, to decrease the distance from pivot point to distal defect.
- Step 2: Develop flap template
  - Templates allow determination of the size, shape and dimension/position of the flap.
  - Use the contralateral normal as a guide to template formation. If not present you can use moulage or additional template formed preoperatively. Many make the template with suture packaging foil.
  - Must replace tissue with exact dimension of template.
    - Flap too large→ Tissue displaced laterally with loss of surface detail.

Division of Maxillofacial Oncology and Reconstructive Surgery, Department of Oral and Maxillofacial Surgery, John Peter Smith Hospital, 1500 South Main Street, Fort Worth, TX 76104, USA
* Corresponding author.
E-mail address: Danielhammeroms@gmail.com

Atlas Oral Maxillofacial Surg Clin N Am 28 (2020) 23–28
1061-3315/20/Published by Elsevier Inc.
https://doi.org/10.1016/j.cxom.2019.11.003

Table 1 Clinical examination components and their significance

Clinical Examination Component	Significance
History	
Etiology and duration of defect	Must ensure wound is stable with proper disease control (clear margins, resolved infection, etc). Recent injury can lead to enlarged defects from edema and gravity. Older wound sites can be contracted leading to underestimating defect size.
Patient risk factor—smokers	Consider smoking cessation before surgery. May elect for delayed flap transfer (most distal aspect of flap is incised 3 months before flap transfer to develop robust distal vasculature). May limit thinning of distal flap during flap transfer.
Patient risk factor—scar near the donor site	Transverse scars overlying the supratrochlear artery are most concerning. Use Doppler imaging to confirm blood supply. Could consider a 3-stage procedure.
Patient risk factor—eyewear	Have postoperative plan to ensure patient can maintain activities of daily living and provide self-care if they are not wearing their glasses.
Patient risk factor—history of head and neck radiation	Obtain a history of location and consider multistage surgery.
Patient risk factor—inability to tolerate staged procedure	Provide patient with previous case photos and consider alternative reconstruction options if necessary.
Physical examination	
Is there a nasal lining and/or cartilage defect?	Additional staged procedure to include cartilage graft as a staged procedure. If so, this could be repaired before substructure and cover/skin reconstruction for proper nasal function.
Define subunits involved in defect	If a defect of a central convex subunit is >50%, plan to resect adjacent normal tissue within the subunit and resurface the entire subunit.[1]
Are the central subunits (lips and eyelids) intact?	All have 3-dimensional shape, proportions and outline with distinct symmetry to contralateral side. Outline and contour are more important than skin quality.[2] Reconstruct lip defect before nasal defect to set foundation.
Where is the patient's hairline?	Low hairlines or short foreheads with previous surgery may require tissue expansion before surgery.
Are there any bony defects contributing to the nasal defect?	If the cheek and lip are not well supported, the nasal reconstruction will not be predictable. The bony substructure must be addressed before the surface. Consider a computed tomography scan to fully understand the underlying bony support.

    - ■ Flap too small→ Contracture with collapse of underlying structure.
- Step 3: Transfer template design to donor site (forehead), locate pedicle and confirm dimensions
  - ○ Mark outline of template with inferior base of planned flap at hairline directly over the supratrochlear artery
    - ■ Locating the arterial pedicle
      - Normally lies approximately 1.7 to 2.2 cm lateral to midsaggital plane, which is usually coincident with the medial border of the brow.
      - The pedicle should be no more than 3 mm medial or lateral to a vertical line extending from the medial canthus.[3,4]
      - Can use Doppler imaging, but 8% of intact supratrochlear arteries cannot be identified by Doppler imaging.
      - The supratrochlear artery is superficial to the orbital rim periosteum at its origin and sandwiched between the corrugator and frontalis muscles. The vessel moves superficially as it travels superiorly entering the subcutaneous tissues 3.5 cm above the orbital rim.
  - ○ Pedicle width should be 1.5 cm with the vessel in the middle of the flap
    - ■ Thinner pedicle width→ risk to pedicle viability
    - ■ Thicker pedicle width→ restricts pivot and can cause kinking
- Step 4: Confirm planned flap's arc of rotation before raising the flap
  - ○ Verify the arc of rotation with passive application of gauze or suture measuring from the pivot point below the medial brow to the most distal aspect of the flap on the forehead and then to the most inferior aspect of the recipient site
    - ■ If more length is needed, extend the flap beyond the hairline or extend the pedicle across the brow toward the medial canthus (medial incision is extended and will be discussed later)
- Step 5: Development of paramedian flap
  - ○ Planned incision is made distally through skin, subcutaneous tissues and frontalis muscle. Dissection is carried inferiorly between the frontalis muscle and the pericranium.
    - ■ 1 cm superior to the orbital rim, the dissection is carried subperiosteally to maintain the pedicle (between corrugator and frontalis)
  - ○ May need to release corrugator muscle to allow for increased arc of rotation.

Table 2 Indications for staging

Number of Stages	Indications and Staged Plan[2]
One (island flap)	Only indicated when the patient has a compromised medical history and cannot have multiple anesthetics or when the patient desires 1 surgery and knows of the aesthetic compromise of a single-stage surgery. A single-stage surgery can lead to excessive bulk, compromised perfusion from overlying tight glabellar skin, and overall poor aesthetic reconstruction.
Two	Ideal for small surface defects of the tip, dorsum or ala that do not require complex support grafts, nasal lining or delicate contour recreation. Stage 1—Flap transfer with *complete* thinning and contouring of distal flap. Stage 2 (3–4 weeks later)—Division and inset of flap without ability to contour distal aspect of flap (tip, ala. and columella). There is a growing amount of literature advocating for stage 2 in 7–10 d after stage 1 with promising results.
Three	Ideal for large, full-thickness defects (including columella and ala). Consider 3 stages for smokers or patients with scars in the region of the flap with concern for blood supply. Stage 1—Flap transfer with minimal thinning and contouring of the distal flap. Stage 2 (3 weeks later)—Entire skin flap is elevated with subdermal plexus remaining with skin and the underlying tissue is contoured. Flap inset with quilting sutures to define alar base, tip contour and dorsal lines. Stage 3 (3 weeks later)—Division and final inset of flap with ability to contour distal aspect of flap (tip, ala and columella)

- Once dissection has reached the level of the brow, only the medial incision should be carried further to determine the pivot point and it should not be extended deeper than papillary dermis to maintain the pedicle.
- Step 6: Management of donor site
  - Wide undermining in the subgaleal plane lateral to donor site defect enables attempt for primary closure in a layered fashion
  - Any area not closed primarily and is inferior to the hairline should be dressed with petroleum gauze and

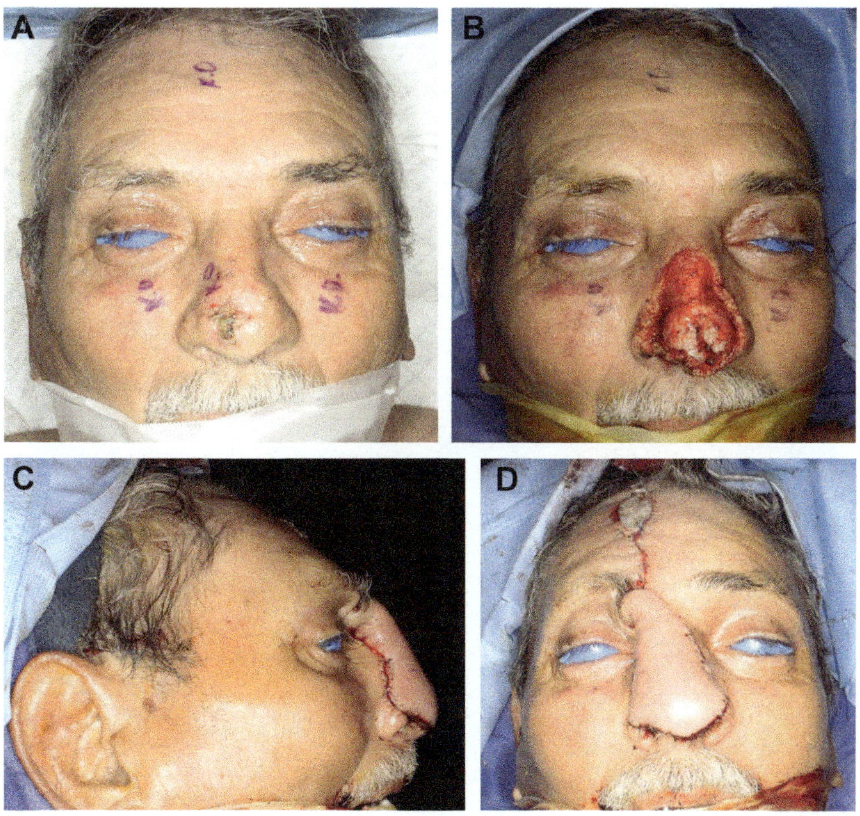

Fig. 1 (*A*) Patient presenting with cutaneous squamous cell carcinoma of the nose. Lesion present on nasal tip, right soft tissue triangle, and right ala. (*B*) After excision of the malignancy with negative margins. Defect now affects bilateral nasal sidewalls, nasal dorsum, nasal tip, bilateral nasal soft tissue triangles, and right alar subunits. (*C*) Profile of paramedian flap after inset. (*D*) Frontal view of inset paramedian forehead flap with split-thickness skin graft placed over the superior flap donor site.

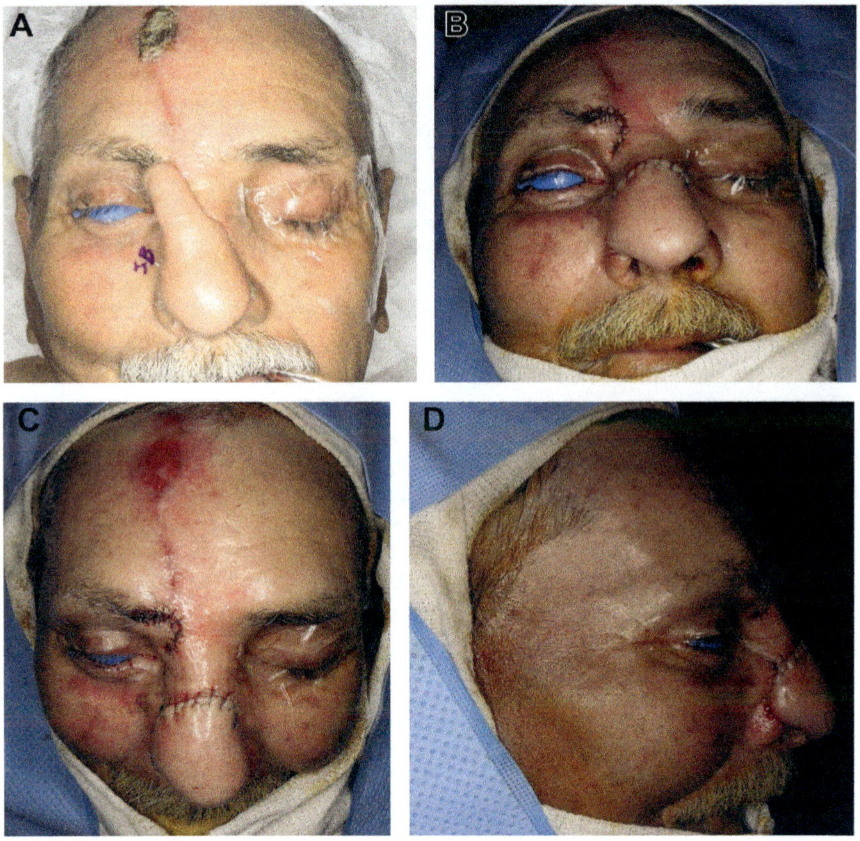

Fig. 2 Patient presenting 3 weeks after harvest and inset of right paramedian forehead flap. (*A*) Patient's presentation on the day of division and inset with a well-vascularized flap and healing skin graft region. (*B*) Frontal view of inset paramedian flap. (*C*) Paramedian flap after division and inset with good color match and contour to surrounding skin and subunits. (*D*) Profile view of inset paramedian flap.

Table 3 The most common complications, and their etiology and management

Complication	Cause	Management
Distal flap necrosis	Inadequate flap dimension (size or bulk) Tension at time of closure Injury to pedicle Excessive re-elevation at time of division and inset	Early debridement and immediate resurfacing limits chance of cartilage infection and preserves substructure. Topical vasodilator.
Infection	Poor sterile technique Necrosis of lining or cartilaginous substructure	Debride and preserve paramedian flap, if possible. If concerned for compromise, return to forehead and allow for infection resolution. If cartilage infection is etiology of infection, elevate flap, debride, and place the patient on proper antibiotics and place new cartilage grafts in 6–8 weeks after resolution.
Poor aesthetic outcome[2]	Categorized as: Minor revision caused by poor landmark definition Major revision caused by failure of dimension, volume, contour, symmetry or function Redo caused by cover and lining deficiency	Minor→ Direct incisions between subunits to enhance landmark definition. Major→ Gross debulking of flap with substructure modification, if needed. Redo→ Second regional flap with excision of previous reconstruction.

allowed to heal secondarily or a split-thickness skin graft can be used (Fig. 1D)

- Step 7: Contouring distal flap
  - The templated region is then debulked with all excess frontalis muscle and subcutaneous tissue removed to enable proper contouring. When given the choice, thin the recipient bed before further thinning of the distal flap.
  - Must keep 2 to 3 mm of subcutaneous tissue on the distal flap to preserve the subdermal plexus. More subcutaneous tissue should be preserved with smokers.
  - Undermine adjacent tissue to defect to avoid trap door defect and establish the nasolabial crease and alar base definition.
- Step 8: Inset of the flap (Fig. 1C, D)
  - Rotate the flap so that the skin is facing the ipsilateral eye limiting the chance of blood draining into the eye
  - Flap is inset to defect site from distal to proximal with a single layer of 5-0 Prolene interrupted sutures
  - If flap blanches, remove sutures in that region and allow to heal secondarily

Stage II (3–4 weeks after flap harvested)

- Step 1: Marking the patient (Fig. 2A)
  - Mark proximal portion of flap with a small inverted "V" to allow for linear closure of the brow
  - Mark the distal portion of flap, which will become the most superior aspect of the flap when inset
- Step 2: Incise planned distal and proximal portion of flap with primary closure of the proximal site
- Step 3: Distal flap inset (Fig. 2B–D)
  - Debulk only cephalic aspect of the distal flap to remove excess subcutaneous tissues, frontalis muscle and scar to create proper contouring. The flap remains vascularized through the distal inset and should not be elevated!
- Step 4: Forehead revision, if needed
  - Excision of scar with bilateral advancement flaps

Potential complications

Complications are rare and when treated promptly have a high propensity to resolve. Table 3 lists the most common complications, and their etiology and management.

Pearls and pitfalls

- Excessive tension at closure can lead to poor perfusion of flap and cause necrosis. Undermine the adjacent skin before inset of flap. If blanching or venous congestion is noted at the time of closure, release the sutures to decrease tension and allow to heal secondarily if needed.
- Avoid thinning the flap significantly in smokers and delay time to division and inset to improve collateral vascular supply. Consider a delayed or 3-stage approach to these patients.
- Always confirm that the template has been properly transferred to the forehead before making any incisions.

Table 4 Clinical results in the literature

Study	Outcomes
The paramedian forehead flap in the reconstruction of nasal defects: 50 consecutive cases[5]	Retrospective analysis of 50 two-staged cases Average defect size was 26 mm Cartilage graft needed in 12% of cases Third stage refinement needed in 4 cases Two patients had postoperative infections resolved with antibiotics Two cases had distal flap necrosis The paramedian forehead flap is reliable with low surgical morbidity and satisfactory aesthetic outcomes
An investigation of patient recorded outcomes following nasal reconstruction with paramedian forehead flaps[6]	Retrospective analysis of 41 one-stage cases 20% of cases required a cartilage graft No flap failures Two patients had postoperative infections that resolved with antibiotics Six patients required second-stage refinement 100% of patients were satisfied with the aesthetic result of their reconstruction The paramedian forehead flap results in low morbidity while yielding very high patient satisfaction rates
Accelerated takedown of the paramedian forehead flap at 1 week: indications, technique, and improving the patient quality of life[7]	Authors were concerned for quality-of-life impairment from an extended period of time between flap transfer and division and inset Retrospective analysis of 26 consecutive patients with accelerated trunk division at a mean of 7.2 days 27% were smokers, 23% were diabetics, and 19% had cartilage grafts used in the reconstruction No patients had flap necrosis 94% of patients preferred division and inset at 1 week, rather than 3 weeks Paramedian forehead flap division and inset at 1 week is safe and effective and can improve quality of life for patients

Immediate postoperative care

- Patient must be instructed on proper care of the flap's "trunk" between harvest and inset.
- No external dressings to the flap because they may compromise flap circulation. Wrap the exposed pedicle in xeroform gauze and apply bacitracin to the incision sites.
- Overnight observation may be warranted if there are concerns for flap viability.
- Prolene sutures are removed 5 to 7 days postoperatively.
- The patient is to not lift anything heavier than 10 pounds for 2 weeks. In addition, they should keep their head elevated and avoid ice application to the flap.
- Recovery from this procedure is usually uneventful with regular clinic follow-up appointments to ensure any postoperative complications are addressed promptly. Ensure the patient is maintaining good wound care, coping with their appearance in the interim, and provide support as needed.

Clinical results in the literature

Table 4 presents clinic results from the literature.

Summary

The paramedian forehead flap is a versatile, dependable flap for complex nasal reconstruction owing to its superior color, texture, size, low morbidity, and good aesthetic result. The procedure can be completed in multiple stages depending on the type of defect and the patient's health and desire outcome. The flap has a very low complication rate and, when complications occur, they can usually be resolved with antibiotics and conservative surgical management.

Disclosure

The authors have nothing to disclose.

References

1. Burger GC, Menick FJ. Subunit principle in nasal reconstruction. Plast Reconstr Surg 1985;76:239.
2. Menick FJ. Nasal reconstruction: art and practice. Philadelphia: Saunders-Elsevier; 2008.
3. Ugur MB, Savranlar A, Uzun L, et al. A reliable surface landmark for localizing supratrochlear artery: medial canthus. Otolaryngol Head Neck Surg 2008;138(2):162–5.
4. Vural E, Batay F, Key JM. Glabellar frown lines as a reliable landmark for the supratrochlear artery. Otolaryngol Head Neck Surg 2000;123(5):543–6.
5. Jones DC. The paramedian forehead flap in the reconstruction of nasal defects: 50 consecutive cases. IJOMS 2011;40:e4.
6. Mughai A, O'Grady K, Kamissetty A, et al. An investigation of patient recorded outcomes following nasal reconstruction with paramedian forehead flaps. BJOMS 2017;55:e120.
7. Somoano B, Kampp J, Gladstone H. Accelerated takedown of the paramedian forehead flap at 1 week: indications, technique, and improving the patient quality of life. J Am Acad Dermatol 2011;65: 97–105.

Further readings

Burget G, Menick F. Aesthetic reconstruction of the nose. St Louis (MO): Mosby; 1993.

Burget GC, Walton R. Optimal use of microvascular free flaps, cartilage grafts and a paramedian forehead flap for aesthetic reconstruction of the nose and adjacent facial units. Plast Reconstr Surg 2007;120: 1228.

MacCarthy J, Lorenc T, Cutting C, et al. The median forehead flap revisited: the blood supply. Plast Reconstr Surg 1985;76:866.

Millard DR. Principalization of plastic surgery. Boston: Little Brown; 1986.

Paddock AC, Frank RW, Spencer HJ, et al. Retrospective chart review of patients who underwent paramedian forehead flap to identify treatment failures and determine contributing factors. Ach Otolaryngol Head Neck Surg 2012;138:367–71.

Reece E, Schaverien M, Rohrich R. The paramedian forehead flap: a dynamic anatomical vascular study verifying safety and clinical implications. Plast Reconstr Surg 2008;121:1956.

Keystone Flap

Kyle S. Ettinger, MD, DDS [a,*], Rui P. Fernandes, MD, DMD, FRCS(Ed) [b], Kevin Arce, MD, DMD [a]

KEYWORDS

• Keystone flap • Perforator flap • Island flap • Advancement flap • Head & neck reconstruction • Maxillofacial surgery

KEY POINTS

- The keystone flap is a random pattern multiperforator-based island advancement flap.
- Perforator-based island flaps derive their blood supply from 1 or multiple vascular perforating branches that emanate from within the central unelevated base of the flap.
- The keystone flap was originally described as 4 types (types I–IV) and numerous subsequent modifications to original keystone flap design have been reported.
- Keystone flap design, application, and elevation are extremely straightforward, presuming that the surgeon possesses a strong foundational knowledge of perforator island flap physiology.
- Keystone flaps have applications for cutaneous reconstruction within the head and neck as well as virtually any other anatomic subsite within the body.

Introduction

When considering reconstruction of cutaneous defects within the head and neck, there often are myriad surgical options available for a given location and size of defect. It remains incumbent on the surgeon to utilize their experience, knowledge base, and skillset to select most appropriate method of reconstruction for a given patient. A fundamental axiom of reconstructive surgery is that local tissue adjacent a surgical defect almost invariably provides the best reconstructive match in terms of tissue quality, thickness, consistency, and color. In this regard, the use of locoregional flaps not only has the potential to reduce operative complexity but also frequently provides more esthetic outcomes compared with other more complicated forms of reconstruction. Maxillofacial surgeons must, therefore, cultivate a broad and diverse knowledge of locoregional soft tissue flaps within their own surgical armamentarium.

The keystone flap is a random pattern multiperforator-based island flap that was originally conceived by Behan[1] in 2003 for repair of cutaneous defects resulting from skin cancer excisions. Although it represents a lesser known local tissue flap within the realm of maxillofacial surgery, it nevertheless holds excellent utility for reconstruction of cutaneous defects within the head and neck.[2–4] The name keystone flap is derived from its semblance to the wedge-shaped keystone of the Roman arch (Fig. 1). The keystone was the critical stone in the Roman arch's construction that was responsible for locking the adjacent stones of the vault into place and redirecting the load of the arch laterally and downward into the adjacent pillars and foundations. Behan's original description of the keystone flap included a classification system that organized flap design into 4 distinct categories (types I–IV), with further subdivision of the type II flap into type IIA and type IIB, depending on whether skin grafting was required to reconstruct the donor site (Fig. 2). Although this classification system loosely correlates with the overall size and relative reconstructive complexity of the surgical defect, from a practical standpoint, having a thorough understanding of the anatomic and physiologic principles of the most basic (type I) keystone flap is all that is needed to understand the basis for the remaining flap subtypes.

Basic island perforator flap anatomy and physiology

As discussed previously, Behan's original description of the keystone flap was that of a multiperforator-based random pattern island advancement flap. Due to the fact that this type of flap is islanded through a circumferential incision that fully interrupts the subdermal plexus from the surrounding tissue, the flap must, therefore, derive its blood supply from one or multiple perforating vessels extending through a broad subcutaneous bed lying directly beneath the flap. This broad subcutaneous bed also must, by necessity, remain adherent to the deeper fascia and underlying muscular bed so as not to disrupt the septocutaneous and musculocutaneous perforators that are emanating from these deeper layers to nourish the overlying skin island (Fig. 3). For the basic keystone flap design, these underlying perforators are never skeletonized or identified during flap mobilization,

[a] Section of Head & Neck Oncologic Surgery and Reconstruction, Division of Oral and Maxillofacial Surgery, Department of Surgery, Mayo Clinic and Mayo College of Medicine, Mail Code: RO_MA_12_03E-OS, 200 First Street Southwest, Rochester, MN 55905, USA
[b] Division of Head and Neck Surgery, Department of Oral and Maxillofacial Surgery, University of Florida College of Medicine – Jacksonville, 653-1 West 8th Street 2nd FL/LRC, Jacksonville, FL 32209, USA
* Corresponding author.
E-mail address: ettinger.kyle@mayo.edu

Atlas Oral Maxillofacial Surg Clin N Am 28 (2020) 29-42
1061-3315/20/© 2019 Elsevier Inc. All rights reserved.
https://doi.org/10.1016/j.cxom.2019.10.001

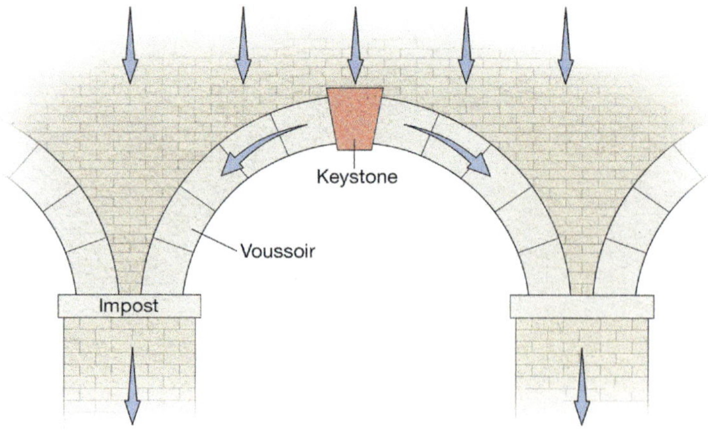

© MAYO CLINIC

Fig. 1 Architectural depiction of a Roman arch with keystone position highlighted.

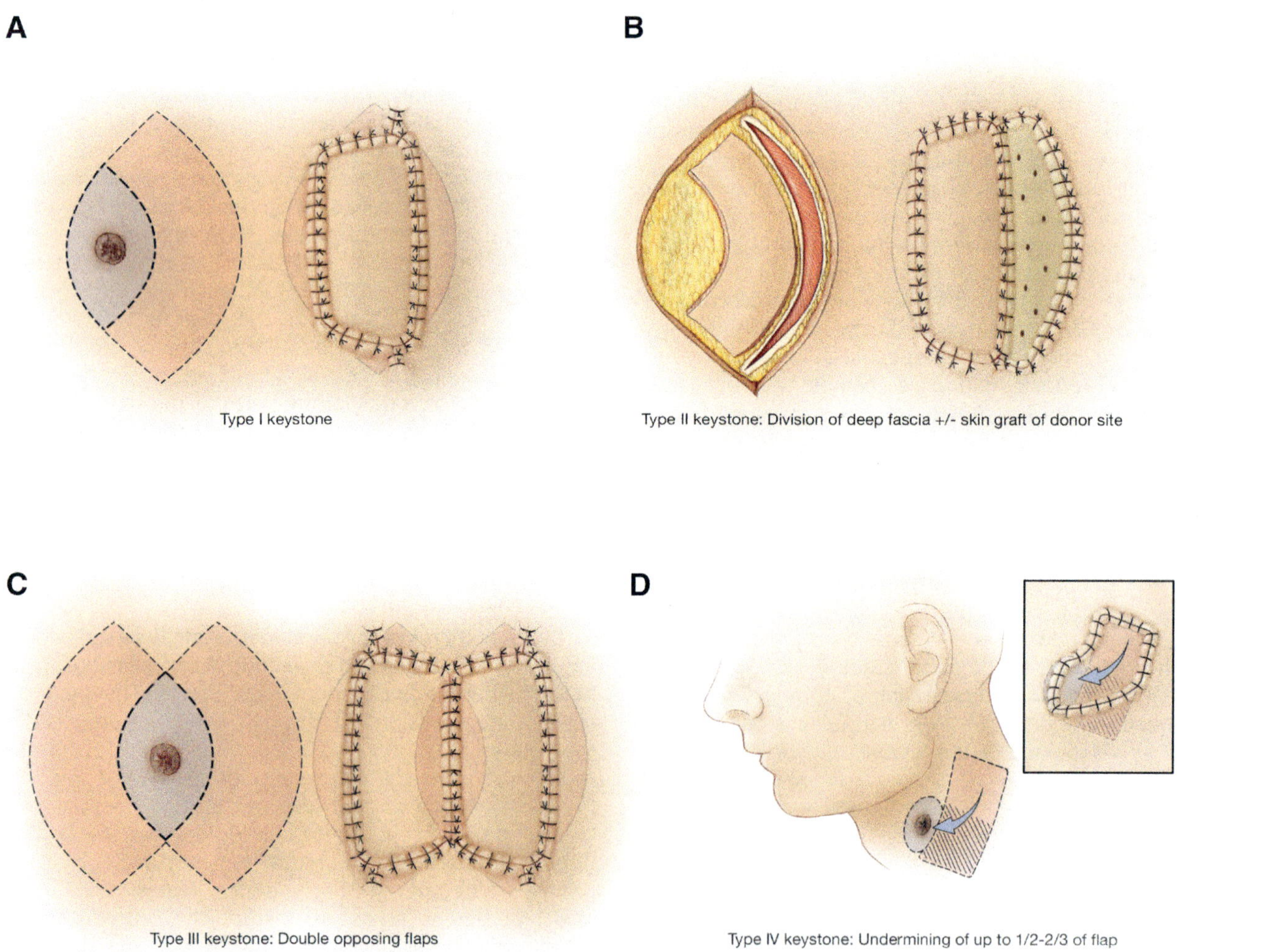

© MAYO CLINIC

Fig. 2 Original types I to IV keystone flap design as described by Behan.[1] (*A*) Type I keystone flap with skin incision only. (*B*) Type II keystone flap with division of the deep fascia along the greater curvature of flap, with or without skin grafting for closure of the donor site. (*C*) Type III keystone flap composed of double opposing keystone flaps. (*D*) Type IV keystone flap with undermining of up to one-half to two-thirds of the flap for advancement and rotation into the defect site.

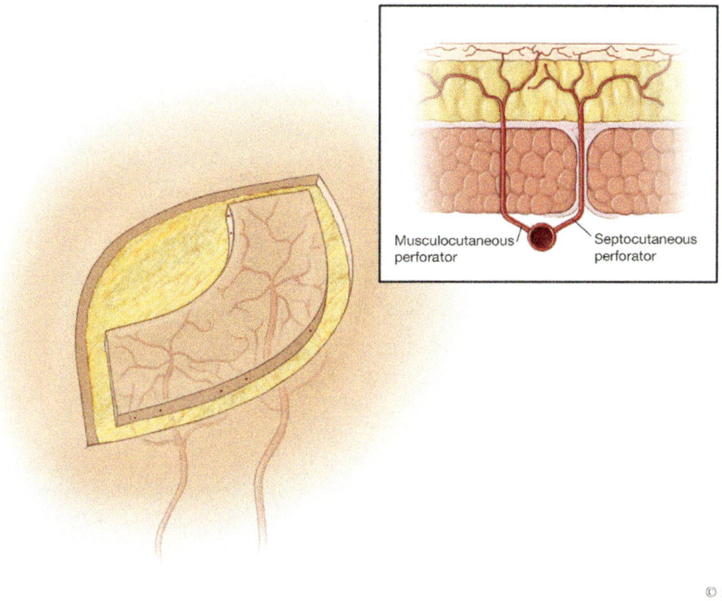

Fig. 3 Depiction of underlying septocutaneous and musculocutaneous perforators supplying vascularity to the keystone flap skin island after circumferential skin and subcutaneous fat incision. Inset box demonstrates the course septocutaneous and musculocutaneous perforators supplying overlying skin.

which is what enables this flap to be elevated safely and quickly—presuming strict adherence to sound surgical/anatomic principles. To ensure that an adequate density of perforators is captured within the flap, Behan has frequently recommended the use of a dermatomal roadmap for keystone flap design.[1,5] In this manner, the planned excision of the primary lesion is oriented such that the long axis of the fusiform excision parallels the regional dermatomal distribution. This excision design and the resulting keystone flap orientation increase the probability of centering the flap within an area of concentrated musculocutaneous and septocutaneous perforators. This methodology assures adequate flap viability without the need for directly identifying underlying perforators with Doppler localization or other methods. By convention, dermatomal segments run longitudinally within the upper and lower extremities and transversely within the chest, abdomen, and pelvis (Fig. 4).[6,7] Due to the rich vascularity within the tissues of the head and neck, strict adherence to this dermatomal orientation of keystone flap design generally is less important compared with reconstruction of defects involving the truncal or appendicular regions of the body. The intrinsic vascularity of the head and neck, however, does not absolve the surgeon from encompassing a sound knowledge of anatomy and fundamental understanding of flap physiology when keystone flaps are used for head and neck reconstruction.

Keystone flap classification and design

As discussed previously, Behan's original description of the keystone flap subdivided its design into 4 distinct types (I–IV) with further subdivision of the type II flap.[1] The basic premise of keystone flap design and execution is understood most readily with the type I flap, because the remaining flap subtypes can be easily extrapolated from the type I design. The following is a basic description of the 4 originally described types of keystone flaps.

Type I

After excision of the primary lesion in a fusiform fashion, a keystone flap is designed adjacent the surgical defect with a 1:1 ratio between the width of the defect and the width of the flap (Fig. 5). Choosing the side of the defect with a greater intrinsic soft tissue laxity aids in mobilization of the flap during the later stages of closure. Note that the short straight limbs of the keystone flap extending off of the terminal points of the fusiform excision are made at 90° angles (see Fig. 5). Once the flap is designed, a skin incision is created circumferentially and deepened into the subcutaneous tissue. There should be minimal undermining beneath the central base of the flap, because this ensures capture of the greatest number of undisturbed perforators within the flap. In the process of undermining the tissues surrounding the keystone flap, care is taken to preserve any superficial veins or nerves coursing across or into the flap itself. The preservation of the superficial venous drainage system augments the venous outflow of the flap whereas preservation of cutaneous nerves allows for a sensate reconstruction. Once the circumferential tissue dissection is performed to the level of the underlying deep fascia, the dissection of the flap is complete. The hallmark of the type I keystone flap is that the entirety of the deep fascia remains intact circumferentially. Flap closure then commences with the terminal portions of the flap being closed in a V-Y fashion (see Fig. 5). This increases the tissue laxity across the central portion of the flap and thus enables primary closure of the ablative defect and the donor site simultaneously (see Fig. 5).

Type II

The type II keystone flap is designed in an identical fashion to the type I flap, with all steps proceeding as described previously. In circumstances in which additional flap mobilization is required to attain primary closure of the defect and donor site, however, the deep fascia is incised along the outer curvilinear

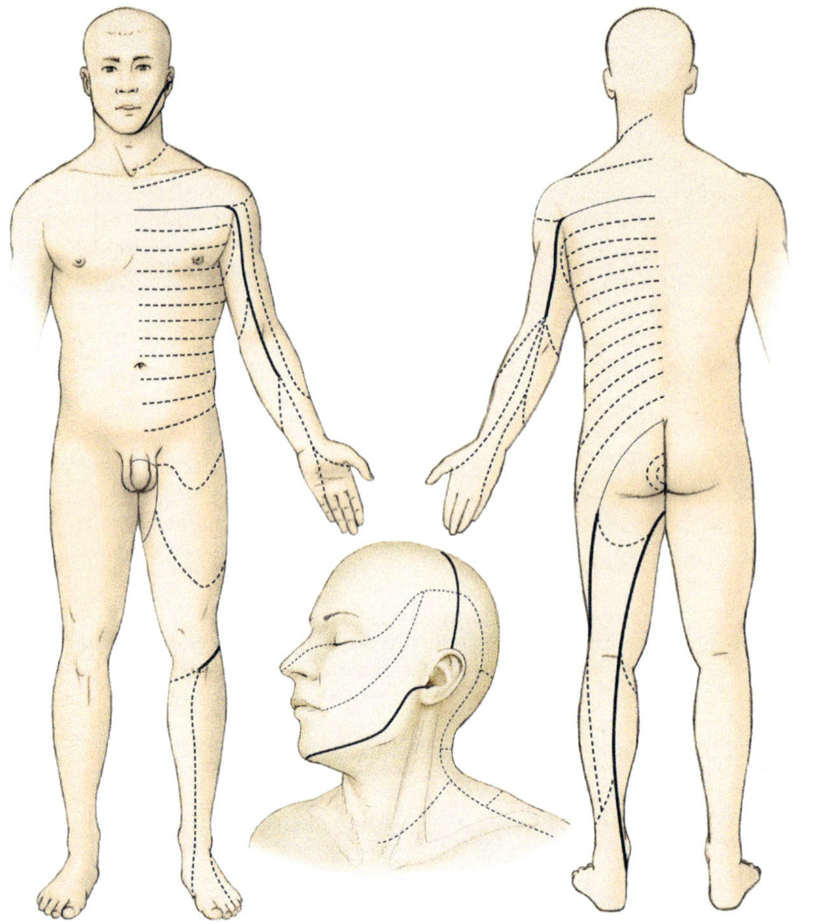

Fig. 4 Orientation of dermatomal segments throughout the body.

margin of the flap (Fig. 6). This additional fascial release enables further mobilization of the keystone flap into the defect while keeping the perforators located in the central portion of the flap intact. The type II keystone flap is further subclassified into types IIA and IIB based on whether or not a skin graft is required to reconstruct the secondary donor site defect (see Fig. 6). Typically, skin grafting of the donor site is necessary in circumstances in which excessive skin tension persists during closure despite typical flap mobilization and subsequent fascial release, as described previously. It bears mentioning at this juncture that an alternative method for eliminating the need for skin grafting involves increasing the width of the keystone flap so that it exceeds the typical 1:1 ratio with the ablative defect (2:1, 3:1, 4:1, and so forth) (see Fig. 18). This specific keystone flap modification is discussed later.

Type III

The type III keystone flap is essentially composed of 2 opposing keystone flaps designed around a central surgical defect (Fig. 7). The type III keystone flap is particularly useful for reconstructing larger ablative defects or defects that are located in areas of the body with low intrinsic soft tissue laxity. Due to the natural laxity of tissues within the face and neck, however, this specific type of keystone flap configuration is not commonly used for head and neck reconstruction. Further impeding its use within the head and neck is the reconstructive principle of camouflaging incisions within relaxed skin tension lines and natural anatomic subunit boundaries of the face in order to minimize visible scarring. The difficulty in attempting to camouflage the incision lines of double opposing keystone flaps within the face can be appreciated, given the inherent geometric complexity of the flaps' design.

Type IV

The type IV keystone flap, as originally described by Behan, is a keystone flap with up to one-half to two-thirds of its subcutaneous base undermined in order to facilitate rotation and/or advancement into an adjacent surgical defect (Fig. 8).[1,3] The vascular supply to the type IV flap originates from perforators arising within the unelevated portion of the flap, which by design are providing vascular supply to the elevated tip of the flap through both the subdermal plexus and suprafascial adipose tissue plexus. In the primary author's opinion, the type IV keystone flap represents a stark departure from the standard flap design and elevation principles that define the hallmark types I to III keystone flaps. Although the successful execution of a type IV keystone flap is certainly founded on the same basic anatomic vascular principles as those of the standard keystone flap, it represents nothing more than a random pattern multiperforator-based pedicled island flap. Although Behan's original description of the type IV flap still incorporated the overall keystone shape to the flaps design, this strict keystone shape no longer is requisite when significant undermining for the advancement/rotation is required to gain

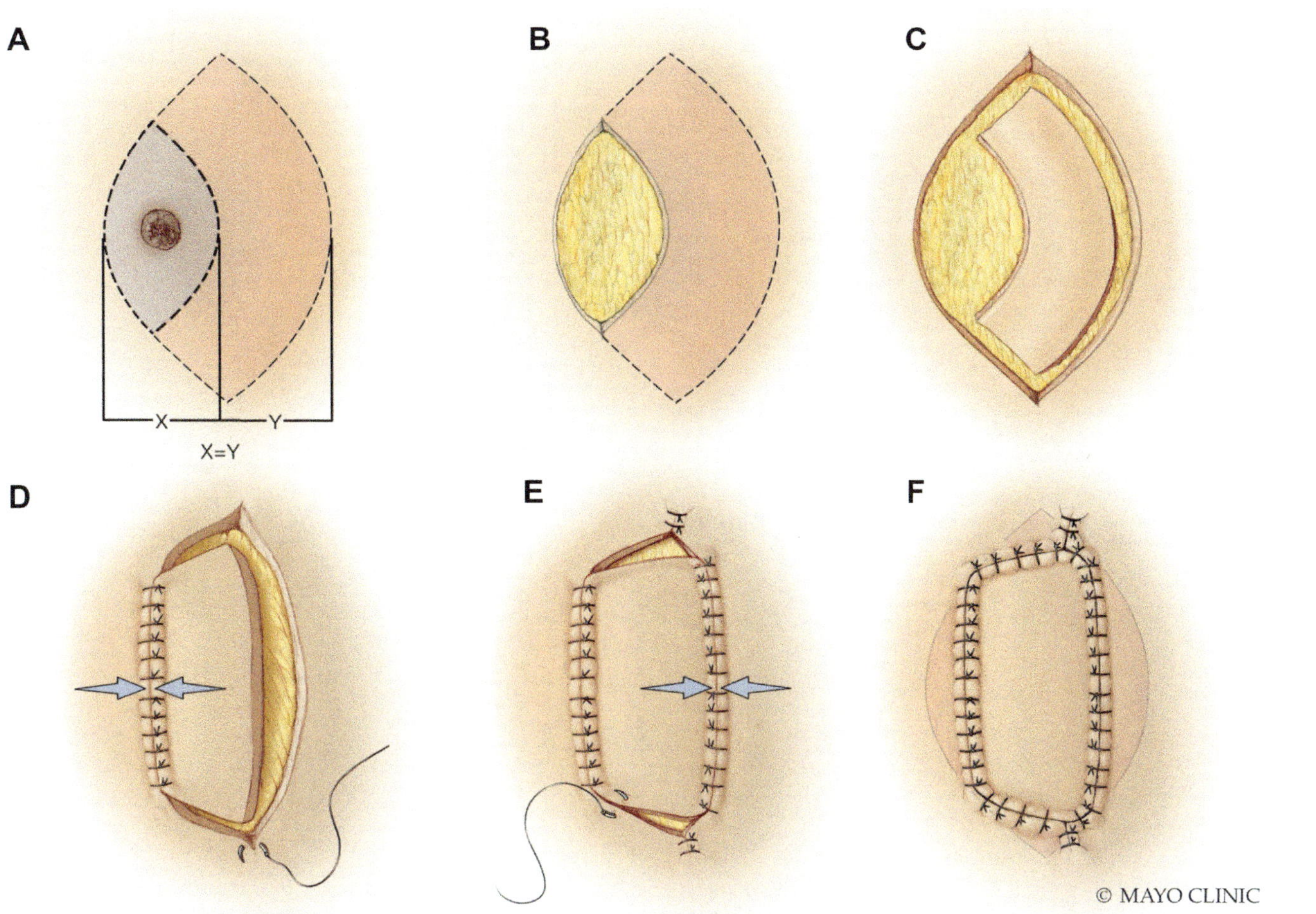

Fig. 5 Stepwise depiction of keystone flap design, elevation, and closure. (*A*) Type I keystone flap design with defect-to-flap ratio of 1:1. Note the short straight limbs of the flap extend from the terminal ends of the fusiform excision at 90° angles. (*B*) Keystone flap design after excision of primary tumor. (*C*) Complete islanding of flap with peripheral subcutaneous dissection performed. (*D–F*) Progressive closure of ablative skin defect and the flap donor site. Note the V-Y closure occurring at the terminal portions of the flap allowing for advancement and reduced tension across the central portion of the flap.

closure. In these circumstances, surgeons may just as easily deviate from the standard keystone configuration and instead choose an alternative flap design, such as fusiform, ovoid, or other geometric pattern, based on the requirements of the ablative defect.[1,6]

Preoperative planning

There are no specific preoperative studies that are required prior to performance of keystone flap reconstruction. It remains a sound operative practice for the surgeon to have preemptively identified how the primary tumor will be resected and how the keystone flap will be designed prior to entering into the operating theater. This planning also should incorporate a well-established plan to accommodate any ablative defect enlargement required to obtain oncologically clear margins and modifications to flap design (increasing the flap to defect width ratio, progressive incision/release of deep fascia, adjunctive need for secondary skin grafting, and so forth) as well as the possibility of selecting an alternative method of local or regional flap reconstruction.

Relative to planning of keystone flap design, surgeons can rely on either the dermatomal roadmap, as previously described by Behan[1] or, alternatively, a handheld Doppler localization of perforators adjacent to the surgical defect. Perforator localization via handheld Doppler frequently is unnecessary, however, for routine types I to III keystone flaps where there is no disruption to the underling broad subcutaneous base of the flap. This is especially true within the head and neck, where a rich vascular network with extensive collateralization exists almost universally. Furthermore, in areas where dominant axial septocutaneous or musculocutaneous perforators are not present, the handheld Doppler does not always return an audible signal, even though a sufficient density of small random perforators exist within the flap base that would adequately sustain the projected skin island. In this circumstance, a novice surgeon may be unnecessarily deterred if relying solely on Doppler corroboration of adequate flap vascularization—a fact that only underscores the importance of the surgeon possessing a commanding knowledge of the fundamental anatomic vascular principles of keystone flaps and perforator-based island flaps in general.

Preparation and patient positioning

No specific patient preparation or positioning is required beyond that which would normally be used to adequately

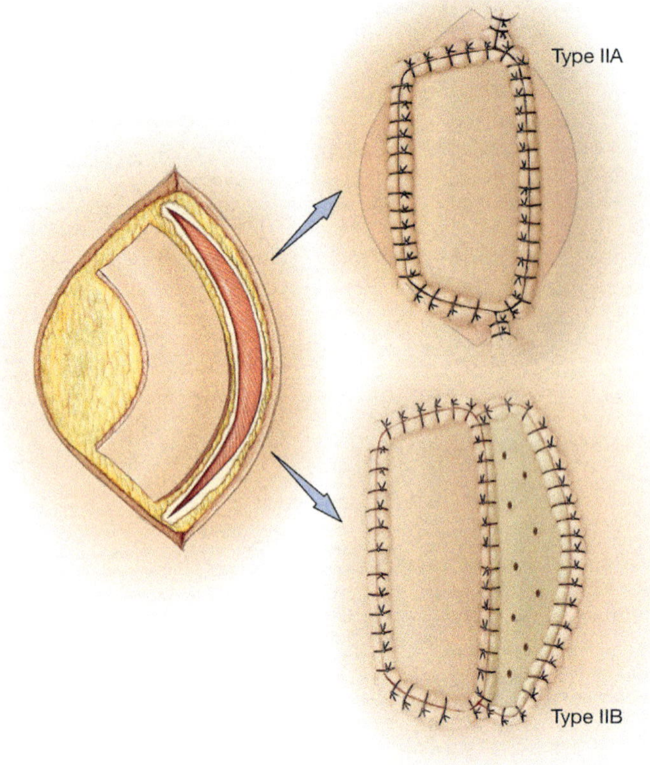

Fig. 6 Depiction of the type II keystone flap. Note the division of the deep fascia along the greater curvature of the flap, allowing for increased mobility for advancement and closure. The type II flap is then further subdivided into type IIA and type IIB, depending on whether or not skin grafting is required for closure of the donor site.

resect the primary tumor and provide sufficient access to adjacent tissue for keystone flap design and elevation.

Surgical approach/procedure

In this case example, a type I keystone flap is demonstrated for the reconstruction after resection of a left temporal cutaneous melanoma (Fig. 9).

Step 1—the surgical field should be prepped and draped in a manner consistent to allow for broad exposure of the soft tissue lesion as well as the anticipated area of the keystone flap itself (Fig. 10).

Step 2—the resection should be designed around the lesion to attain wide oncologic clearance of the tumor with negative margins (Fig. 11). Note that although Behan's original keystone flap description[1] recommended for a

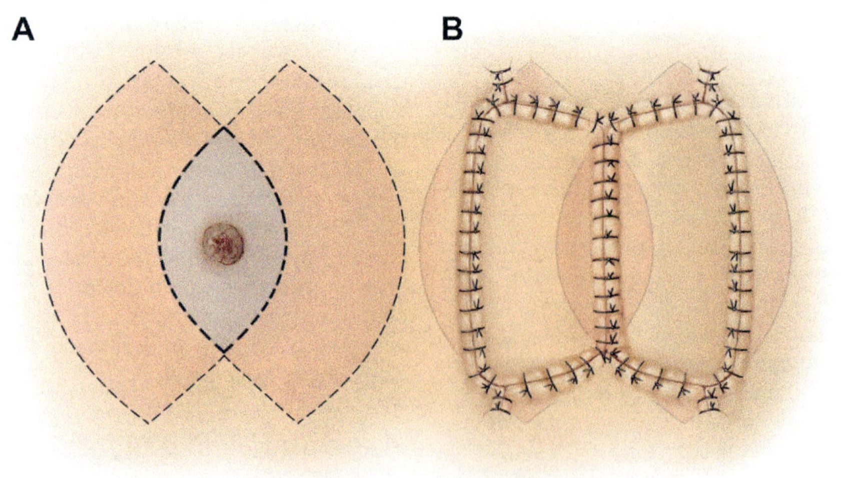

Fig. 7 The (*A*) design and (*B*) closure of the type III double opposing keystone flap.

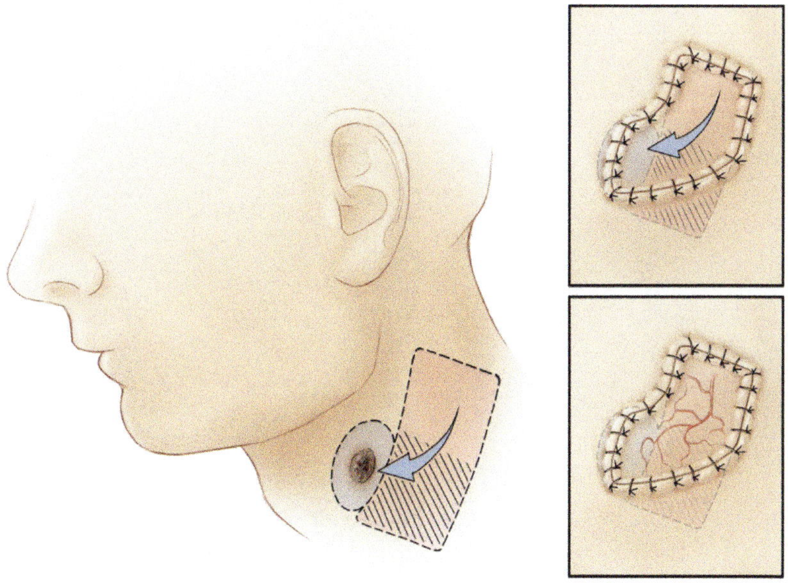

© MAYO CLINIC

Fig. 8 Depiction of the type IV keystone flap with up to one-half to two-thirds of the flap being undermined. Figure insets depict the advancement and rotation of the undermined portion of the flap (upper inset) as well as the vascularization of the flap emanating from the unelevated base of the flap and nourishing the tip through the subdermal plexus and suprafascial adipose plexus (lower inset).

fusiform excision, this is not mandatory and other forms of excision geometry can be employed with equivalent effect.

Step 3—on verification of negative resection margins, the keystone flap is designed with 90° angles extending of the terminal portions of the excision and with a defect–to-flap–width ratio of 1:1 (Fig. 12).

Step 4—perform circumferential incision of the flap through skin, dermis, and subcutaneous fat down to the level of the underlying deep fascia (Fig. 13). Note that in this anatomic region of the head and neck, the fascia immediately deep to the subcutaneous fat is the temporoparietal fascia, which is the fascial layer that houses the primary vascular pedicle supplying the flap—the superficial temporal artery and vein. Unique to this dissection, care would be taken to preserve the integrity of the superficial temporal vessels along the margin of the flap where these vessels are coursing so as not to devascularize the skin island. Note that the anterior branch of the superficial temporal artery is seen coursing obliquely across the resection defect (see Fig. 13).

Step 5—the flap is then checked for adequate mobility to allow for primary closure of the ablative defect and donor site. If inadequate flap mobility is not obtained, the deep fascia along the greater curvature of the flap can be incised to increase advancement into the ablative defect (Fig. 14). Note that with the existing flap orientation and design, the incision of the deep fascia along the greater

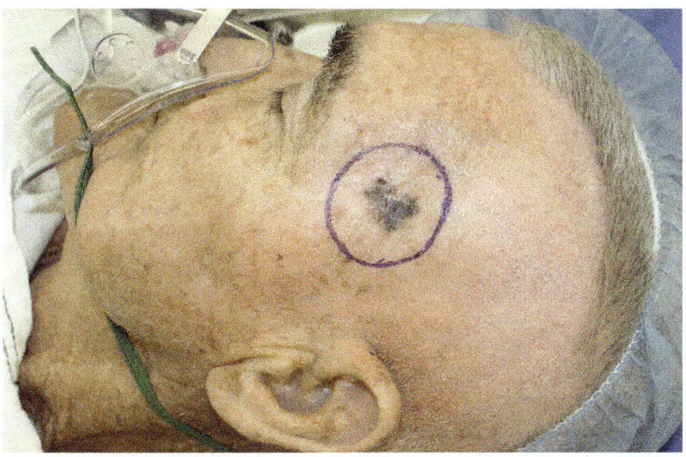

Fig. 9 Left temporal cutaneous melanoma with preoperatively planned excision margin (blue circle).

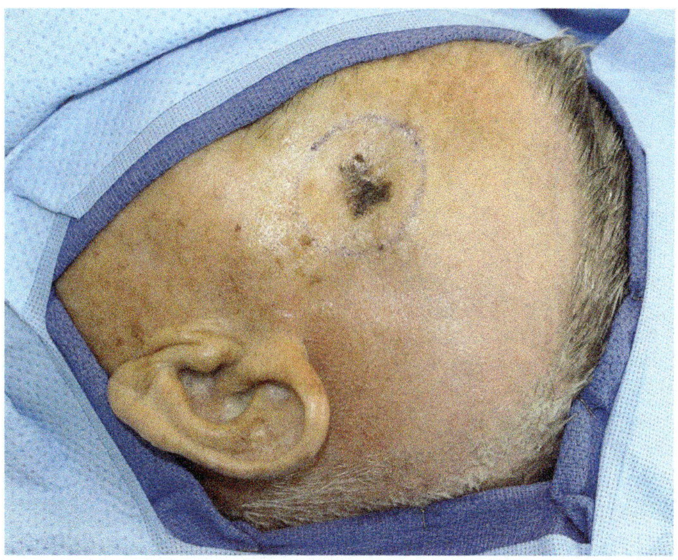

Fig. 10 Prepping and draping of surgical field to accommodate tumor resection and keystone flap elevation.

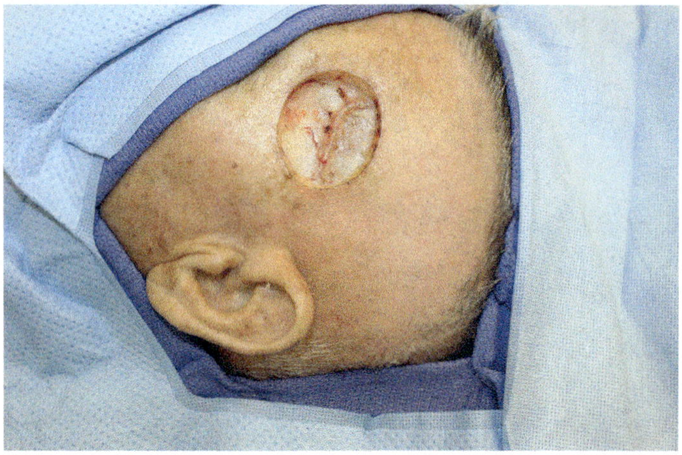

Fig. 11 Resection of primary tumor with oncologically negative margins.

curvature does not compromise the proximal vascular pedicle of the flap (see Fig. 14).

Step 6—once adequate flap mobility is achieved, closure commences in the typical fashion with interrupted deep dermal suturing followed by closure of the skin (Fig. 15). Although Behan's original description of the keystone flap went into extensive detail on flap closure utilizing a continuous horizontal everting mattress suture technique,[1] the authors have not found this necessary in practice and a standard closure, as described previously, yields excellent clinical results (Fig. 16). Occasionally, it is advantageous to not begin closure at the central portion of the defect but rather to begin at the periphery, because this allows for progressive tissue advancement into the central portion of the defect and minimizes the wound tension progressively. It also should be noted that flap closure occasionally involves excision of specific portions of the flap to eliminate standing cones (colloquially, dog ears) and to remove areas of flap redundancy. This most often is necessary in the areas of the 90° angles along the lesser curvature of the flap, as depicted in Fig. 17.

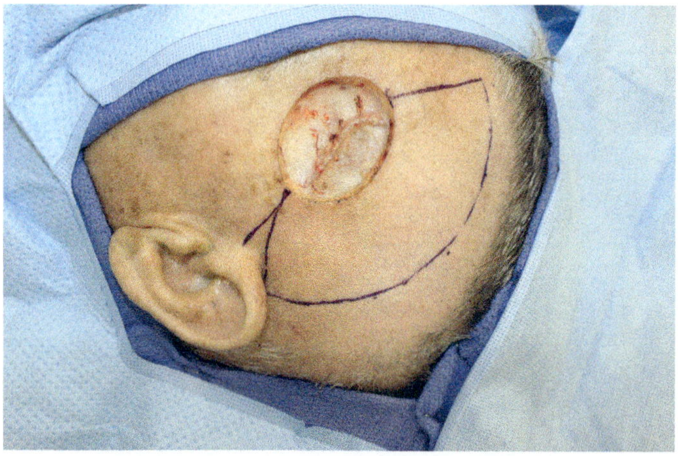

Fig. 12 Type I keystone flap design with 1:1 flap width-to-defect ratio. Note the area of skin at the superior margin of the helix that will be excised to facilitate closure.

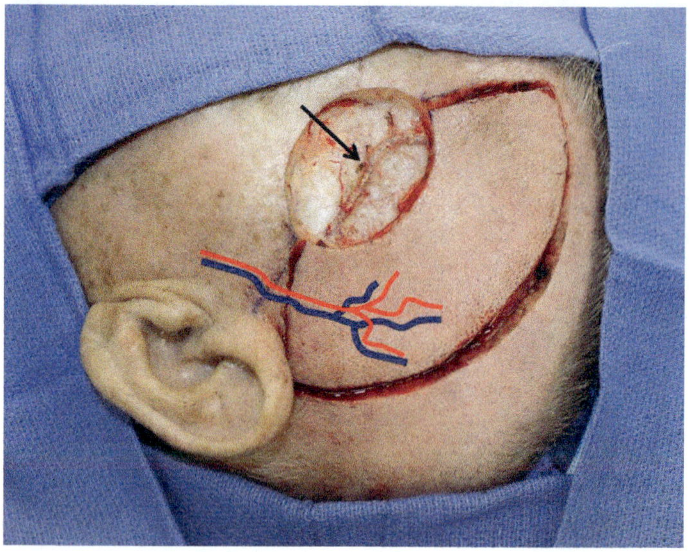

Fig. 13 Keystone flap circumferentially islanded to the level of the underlying fascia (temporoparietal fascia). The takeoff and ramification of the superficial temporal vessels are diagrammed on the photo. Care would be taken during dissection along this margin of the flap so as not to disrupt the continuity of these vessels that are supplying the skin island. The arrow denotes the anterior branch of the superficial temporal artery coursing across the resection defect.

Immediate postoperative care and recovery

Postoperative care for keystone flaps is no different from that of any other local flap used within the head and neck. Daily care should consist of frequent cleansing of incision lines and regular application of a petrolatum based ointment to

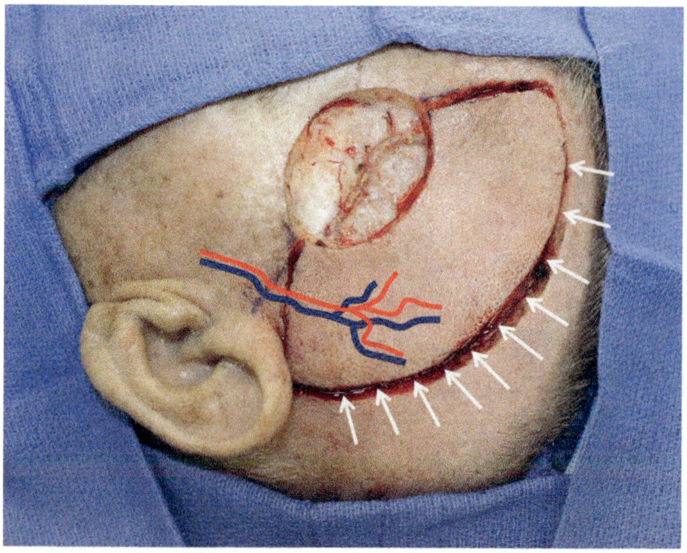

Fig. 14 To improve flap mobility the fascia immediately deep to the skin island (temporoparietal fascia) can be incised along the greater curvature of the flap (*arrows*). Incising the deep fascia in this region does not compromise the primary vascular pedicle of the flap. This highlights the importance of preemptively anticipating the need for flap modifications and incorporating that into the preoperative flap design to ensure adequate flap vascularity.

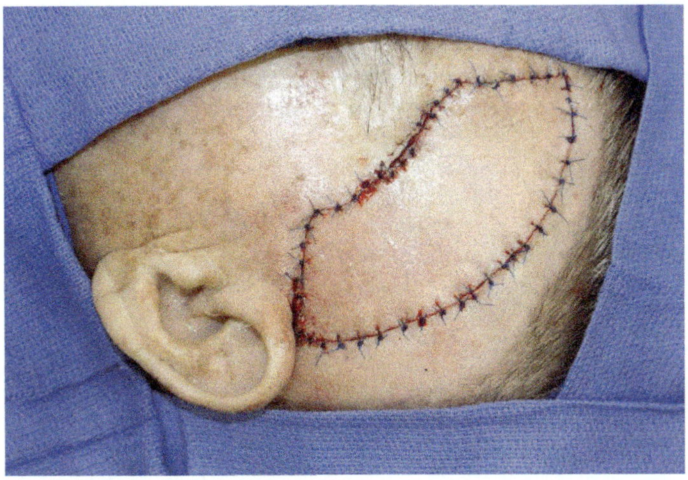

Fig. 15 Layered closure of the ablative defect and the keystone flap donor site.

facilitate incisional wound healing. After keystone flap reconstruction, patients frequently have minimal pain due to the limited nature of the dissection and the temporary denervation of cutaneous inputs to the flap through skin islanding. Nonabsorbable sutures for skin closure should be removed within 5 days to 10 days in order to minimize unaesthetic epithelization along suture tracts; however, exact timing of suture removal always should be contingent on the native soft tissue laxity and degree of wound healing at the anticipated time of removal. Although periods of immobilization occasionally are necessary for adequate healing of keystone flaps used for trunk or extremity defects, periods of immobilization or prolonged activity restrictions are largely unnecessary for keystone flap reconstruction within the head and neck.

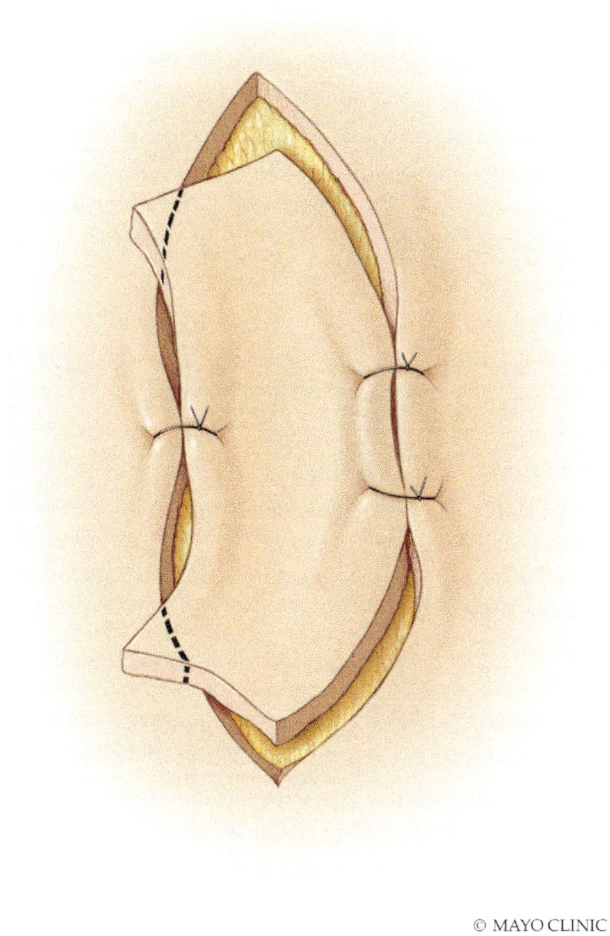

Fig. 17 Depiction of partial closure of keystone flap with demarcation along redundant areas of the flap that are commonly trimmed in order to facilitate insetting.

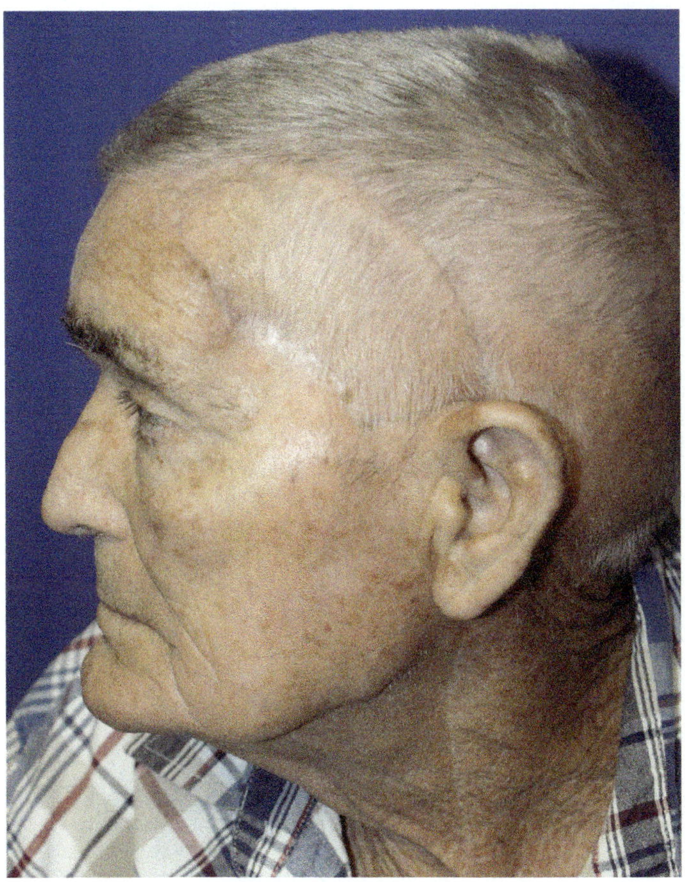

Fig. 16 Early postoperative healing of type I keystone flap.

Potential complications

As with all local soft tissue flaps, disregard for basic vascular physiology can lead to partial or even total flap necrosis, which can greatly compromise the reconstructive outcome. Execution of the keystone flaps is an extremely straightforward proposition, however, for the surgeon who possesses a thorough understanding of the underlying vascular principles that maintain the viability of perforator island flaps. With reliance on appropriate patient selection coupled with sound surgical technique during flap elevation, mobilization, and closure, the expected major complication rate for keystone flaps (ie, partial or total flap necrosis) should be less than 10%.[6] Minor complications, including incisional dehiscence or delayed wound healing, can be treated easily with conservative local wound care measures.

Pearls and pitfalls

As discussed previously, patient selection plays an important role in determining the suitability of keystone flaps for reconstruction of head and neck defects. Caution should be exercised in patients with prior history of surgical skin undermining involving the operative field, patients with irradiated tissue beds, or wounds currently in an inflammatory state, as each of these scenarios compromises flap vascularity and soft tissue laxity.[6] Keystone flaps can certainly be utilized in irradiated and traumatized tissue beds with high expectations for flap success[8,9]; however, surgeons must remain cognizant of the impacts of each of these scenarios on generalized wound healing—regardless of the type of flap reconstruction that is selected.

As discussed previously, there are several modifications to Behan's original description of the keystone flap that have subsequently been reported.[6,7,10–15] Although some of these modifications have sound physiologic basis for improving aspects of the keystone flap technique, others are not as well

Table 1 Modifications to traditional keystone flap design

Technique/Design	Modification	Potential Advantages	Potential Drawbacks
Increased flap-to-defect ratio (2:1, 3:1, 4:1, etc.)[6,7,14]	Flap width is increased beyond the traditional 1:1 flap-to-defect ratio (Fig. 18)	• Incorporation of a larger perforator territory • Increases soft tissue laxity facilitating closure of defect and donor site	• Increased length of surgical incisions and larger donor site area
Extended incision of deep fascia[6,7,14]	The deep fascia is progressively incised to facilitate flap advancement into ablative defect. Near-complete or even total circumferential incision of fascia can be performed based on reconstructive needs (Fig. 19).	• Greatly improves flap advancement without compromising centrally located vascular perforators	• Potential for injuring peripherally located septocutaneous or musculocutaneous perforators if inappropriate surgical technique used (ie, inadvertent dissection deep to the fascia)
Asymmetric limb angulation[6,7,14]	The traditional 90° short straight limbs of keystone flap are intentionally designed asymmetrically or at differing angles (Fig. 20).	• Avoids critical structures or orients incision lines along anatomic subunits/relaxed skin tension lines	• May require differential suturing for closure or additional flap tailoring to achieve optimal reconstructive outcome
Fortune cookie modification[12]	Ablation is performed with circular rather than fusiform excision. Limbs of keystone flap are designed with origins at the margin of the defect most distant from the flap (leaving 2 triangular components along the lesser curvature). The flap apices and margins adjacent the defect are closed linearly with remainder of flap advancement proceeding in traditional fashion (Fig. 21).	• Minimizes need for secondary soft tissue excision • Reduces overall defect size by reliance on circular rather than fusiform excision design	• Can leave standing cone deformity that may require secondary revision
Boat-shaped flap[13]	Flap is designed with a V-shaped modification to the incision along the greater curvature of the flap (Fig. 22). The sail portion of the flap is then undermined if necessary and then closed in a V-Y fashion.	• Theoretically reduces skin tension across the central portion of the defect through the additional flap advancement gained from the V-Y closure	• Central flap undermining has the potential to injure vascular perforators and compromise overall flap vascularity.
Sydney Melanoma Unit modification[15]	Flap is designed with an incomplete incision along the midportion of the greater curvature of the flap. The resulting skin bridge remains intact once the flap is advanced into the ablative defect (Fig. 23).	• Theoretically preserves additional venous and lymphatic outflow through the undisturbed subdermal plexus of the skin bridge	• Skin bridge may impede advancement and obscures underlying deep fascia if additional release is required. • Skin bridge is physiologically unnecessary given perforator island flap physiology and vascularization from centrally located deep perforator vessels.

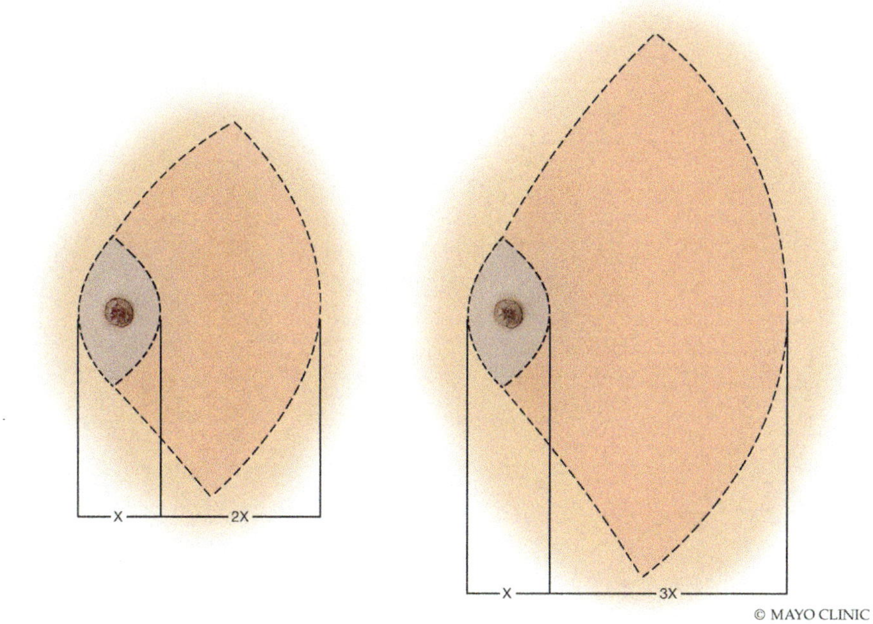

Fig. 18 Depiction of keystone flap designs with increased flap-to-defect ratio. The left panel depicts a 2:1 flap-to-defect ratio and the right panel depicts a 3:1 flap-to-defect ratio.

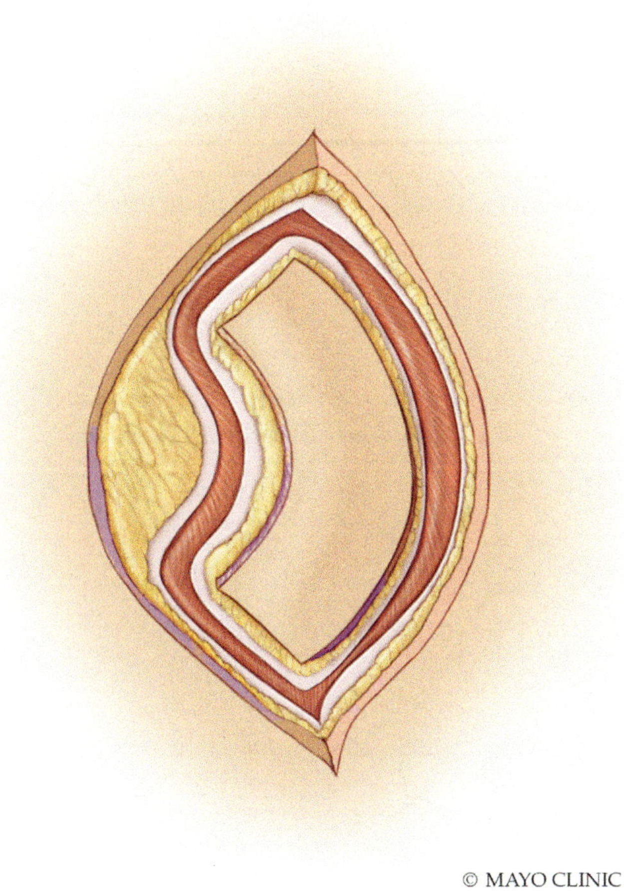

Fig. 19 Depiction of extended circumferential incision of deep fascia to maximize mobilization and advancement of flap. Note that circumferential incision of fascia will not disrupt the centrally located perforators deep to the skin island.

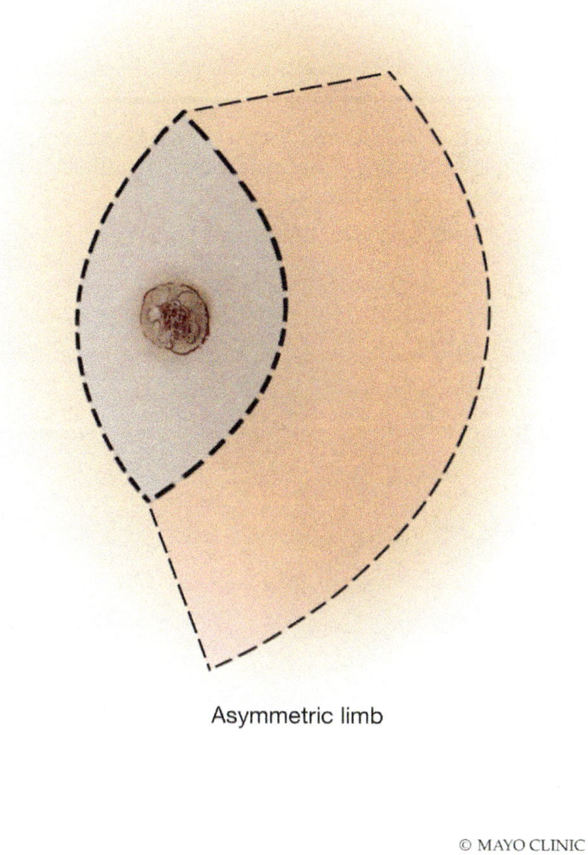

Fig. 20 Depiction of keystone flap design with asymmetric limb angulations. This modification is useful for avoidance of critical structures or reorienting incision lines to fall within anatomic boundaries or relaxed skin tension lines.

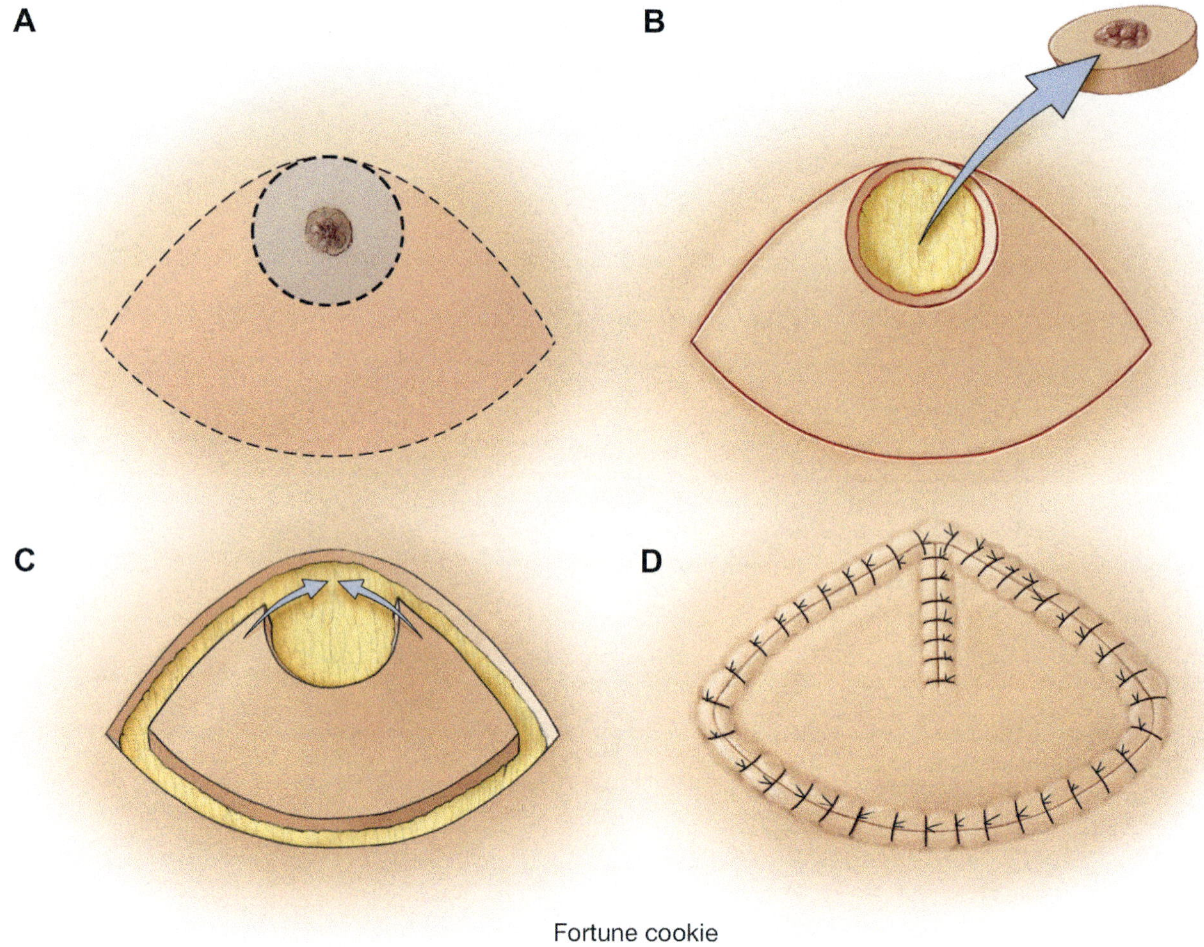

© MAYO CLINIC

Fig. 21 Fortune cookie modification of the keystone flap. (*A*) Flap design. Note the use of a circular resection and the short limbs of the keystone flap originating at the distant margin of the flap rather than the standard origin at the poles of the defect. (*B*) Tumor removal, (*C*) flap dissection, and (*D*) closure.

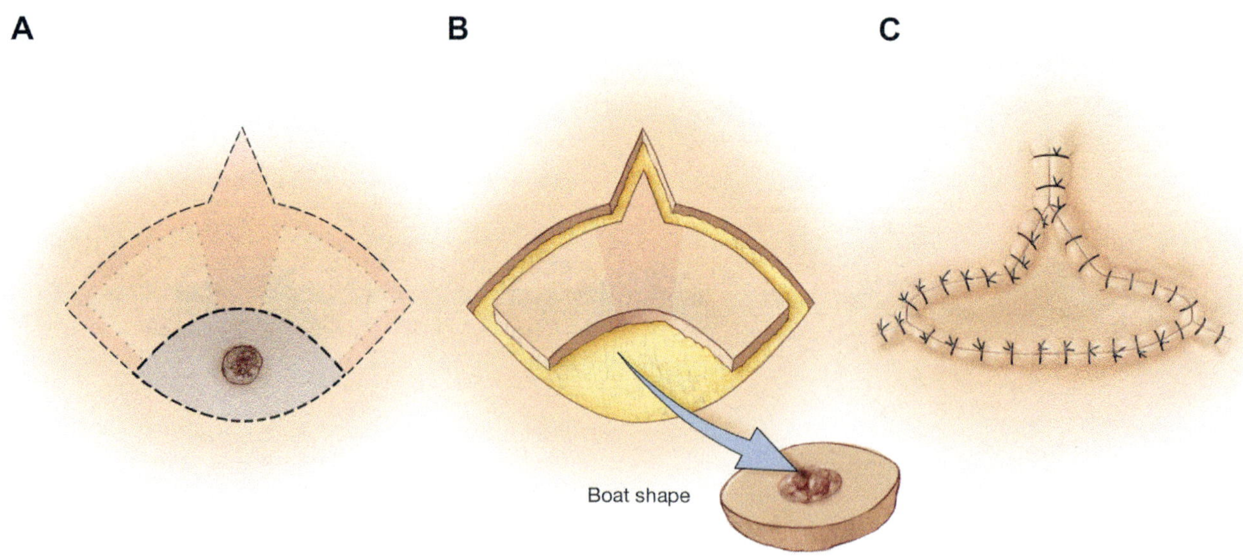

© MAYO CLINIC

Fig. 22 Boat-shaped modification of the keystone flap. (*A*) Flap design. Note the lighter shaded areas correspond to the regions of the flap that are not undermined to preserve underlying perforators, whereas the central sail and mast portion of the flap is undermined in a suprafascial plane. (*B*) Tumor resection with the shaded central portion highlighting the undermined area of the flap. (*C*) Flap advancement and closure with a V-Y closure facilitating advancement at the sail portion of the flap and minimizing the skin deficit in the donor site.

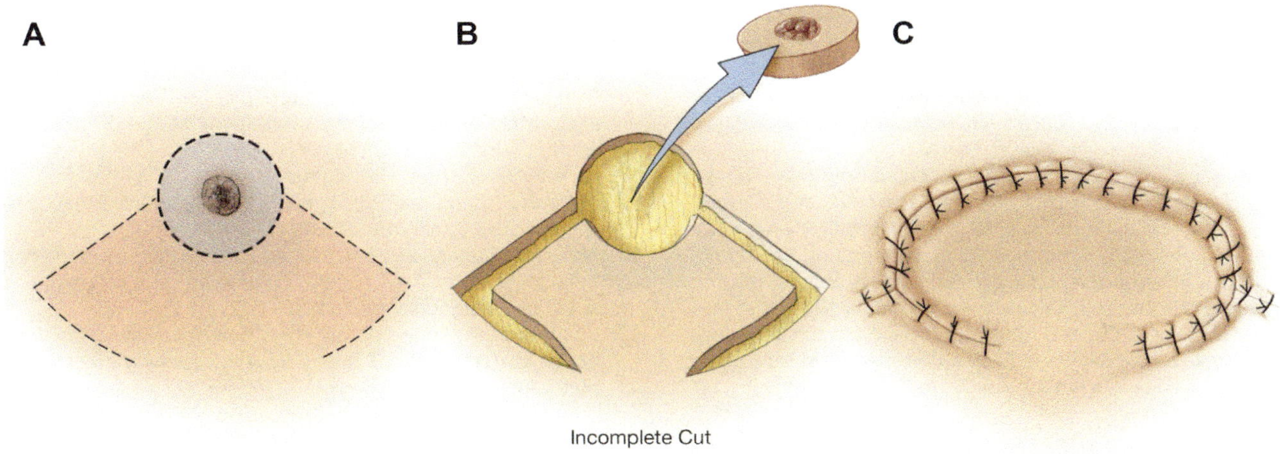

© MAYO CLINIC

Fig. 23 The Sydney Melanoma Unit modification. (*A*) Flap design. (*B*) Flap elevation. Note the incomplete cut along the greater curvature of the flap. (*C*) Closure of the flap.

founded in the purported benefits/improvements on the original flap design and implementation.[5,16] An in-depth discussion regarding the merits and drawbacks of each of these design modifications is beyond the scope of this article; however, synoptic information regarding various keystone flap modifications are depicted in Table 1 and Figs. 18–20.

Clinical results in literature

Since its original description, the keystone flap has demonstrated excellent versatility for local reconstruction of soft tissue defects throughout the body.[1–21] In addition to routine application for small cutaneous defects of the head and neck, the keystone flap has documented success in reconstructing defects within radiated tissue beds,[8] in large composite facial resections for patients ill-suited for free flap reconstruction,[3] and among elderly populations with advanced head and neck cancer.[4] The keystone flap also has been described for reducing donor site morbidity after free flap harvest, specifically enabling primary closure of thigh defects after large anterolateral thigh flap harvests that otherwise would require unsightly split-thickness skin grafting for closure.[17] A recent systematic review demonstrated the exceedingly low failure rates seen with properly executed keystone flap reconstructions. Partial and complete flap failure rates of 1.1% and 0.7% were seen, respectively, among a pooled cohort of 245 patients with 282 keystone flaps performed for lower extremity reconstruction.[21]

Summary

The keystone flap is an excellent, straightforward, and reliable flap for restoring cutaneous defects within the head, neck, and face. As a random pattern multiperforator-based island flap, the keystone flap has excellent reconstructive versatility and can greatly diminish operative complexity, surgical time, and patient morbidity when applied to the appropriate clinical scenario. With an understanding of basic keystone flap physiology, the surgeon can rapidly modify the flap in a multitude of ways in order to suit the specific reconstructive needs of the patient and defect being reconstructed. Maxillofacial surgeons should be aware of this flap as an option for simple and even complex forms of head and neck reconstruction and maintain it as a routine option within their own surgical armamentaria.

Disclosure

The authors have nothing to disclose.

References

1. Behan FC. The keystone design perforator island flap in reconstructive surgery. ANZ J Surg 2003;73(3):112–20.
2. Behan FC, Rozen WM, Wilson J, et al. The cervico-submental keystone island flap for locoregional head and neck reconstruction. J Plast Reconstr Aesthet Surg 2013;66(1):23–8.
3. Behan FC, Lo CH, Sizeland A, et al. Keystone island flap reconstruction of parotid defects. Plast Reconstr Surg 2012;130(1):36e–41e.
4. Behan F, Sizeland A, Gilmour F, et al. Use of the keystone island flap for advanced head and neck cancer in the elderly-a principle of amelioration. J Plast Reconstr Aesthet Surg 2010;63(5):739–45.
5. Behan F, Lo C. Principles and misconceptions regarding the keystone island flap. Ann Surg Oncol 2009;16(6):1722–3.
6. Abraham JT, Saint-Cyr M. Keystone and pedicle perforator flaps in reconstructive surgery: new modifications and applications. Clin Plast Surg 2017;44(2):385–402.
7. Mohan AT, Rammos CK, Akhavan AA, et al. Evolving concepts of keystone perforator island flaps (KPIF): principles of perforator anatomy, design modifications, and extended clinical applications. Plast Reconstr Surg 2016;137(6):1909–20.
8. Behan F, Sizeland A, Porcedu S, et al. Keystone island flap: an alternative reconstructive option to free flaps in irradiated tissue. ANZ J Surg 2006;76(5):407–13.
9. Sliesarenko SV, Badiul PO, Sliesarenko KS. Extensive mine-shrapnel and gunshot wound closure using keystone island perforator flaps. Plast Reconstr Surg Glob Open 2016;4(5):e723.
10. Behan FC, Rozen WM, Lo CH, et al. The omega - Omega - variant designs (types A and B) of the keystone perforator island flap. ANZ J Surg 2011;81(9):650–2.
11. Behan FC, Rozen WM, Tan S. Yin-Yang flaps: the mathematics of two keystone island flaps for reconstructing increasingly large defects. ANZ J Surg 2011;81(7–8):574–5.

12. Byun IH, Kim CW, Park TH. The modified keystone flap for pressure ulcers: a modification of the keystone flap with rotation and advancement. Ann Plast Surg 2019;82(3):299–303.
13. Fang S, Tang W, Li Y, et al. A novel modification of keystone flap for superficial defects repair. J Plast Reconstr Aesthet Surg 2019;72(5): 848–62.
14. Mohan AT, Sur YJ, Zhu L, et al. The concepts of propeller, perforator, keystone, and other local flaps and their role in the evolution of reconstruction. Plast Reconstr Surg 2016;138(4):710e–29e.
15. Moncrieff MD, Bowen F, Thompson JF, et al. Keystone flap reconstruction of primary melanoma excision defects of the leg-the end of the skin graft? Ann Surg Oncol 2008;15(10):2867–73.
16. Donovan LC, Douglas CD, Van Helden D. Wound tension and 'closability' with keystone flaps, V-Y flaps and primary closure: a study in fresh-frozen cadavers. ANZ J Surg 2018;88(5):486–90.
17. Turin SY, Spitz JA, Alexander K, et al. Decreasing ALT donor site morbidity with the keystone flap. Microsurgery 2018;38(6): 621–6.
18. Pelissier P, Santoul M, Pinsolle V, et al. The keystone design perforator island flap. Part I: anatomic study. J Plast Reconstr Aesthet Surg 2007;60(8):883–7.
19. Pelissier P, Gardet H, Pinsolle V, et al. The keystone design perforator island flap. Part II: clinical applications. J Plast Reconstr Aesthet Surg 2007;60(8):888–91.
20. Khouri JS, Egeland BM, Daily SD, et al. The keystone island flap: use in large defects of the trunk and extremities in soft-tissue reconstruction. Plast Reconstr Surg 2011;127(3):1212–21.
21. Huang J, Yu N, Long X, et al. A systematic review of the keystone design perforator island flap in lower extremity defects. Medicine (Baltimore) 2017;96(21):e6842.

Glabellar Flaps for Reconstruction of Skin Defects

Alba Sanjuan-Sanjuan, MD [a], Marek Ogledzki, DMD, MD [a], Carlos A. Ramirez, MD, DDS [b,c,d,*]

KEYWORDS

• Glabellar • Reconstruction • Nasal reconstruction • Dorsal nasal flap • Frontonasal flap • Medial canthal

KEY POINTS

- The glabellar flap can easily be performed, using local skin that is of similar structure, texture, consistency, and color to that of the defect.
- Glabellar area is commonly used for the reconstruction of the upper nasal dorsum or medial canthal area.
- A dorsal nasal flap is a modification of the glabellar flap. It can be used for reconstruction of nasal tip and midnasal wounds.
- The flap may be thinned significantly at the time of harvest, without compromising the circulation to the flap to avoid skin thickness discrepancy.
- Potential complications include widening the limbus owing to tension on the medial canthus, and unwanted pull on the medially situated brow areas.

Introduction

Facial skin defect reconstruction follows both the facial subunits and the "like is used to repair like" principle.[1,2] The absent unit must be replaced with like tissue in regard to quantity and quality, following its pattern, surface area, and contour.[3]

The glabellar area is a source of redundant thick skin that is commonly used for the reconstruction of the upper nasal dorsum and medial canthal area.[4,5] The glabellar flap has been originally described as a V-Y advancement flap, based on random circulation. However, it has been modified in multiple occasions or used in combination with other procedures to reconstruct more distal defects involving the nasal tip, columella, alar lobule, and upper lip.[2,6,7]

The objective of this article is to revisit the use of the glabellar flap and its variations for the reconstruction of defects in the nasal and paranasal area.

Glabellar flap

History

The use of glabellar skin was first reported in 1818 by Carl von Graefe in his book devoted solely to rhinoplasty, "Rhinoplastik." The glabellar flap was then used in the later centuries by many other surgeons. Initially used as a V-Y advancement flap, Field[8] modified it to a transposition "banner" unipedicled flap with the base arising from the contralateral lateral nasal wall. Morrison and colleagues[6] in 1955 described the reverse glabellar flap for distal defects (nasal tip, alar lobule, columella, and even the upper lip) and Seyhan[7] in 2009 used this reverse flap to reconstruct lower eyelid, nose, medial canthal and malar region.

In 1967, Rieger[9] modified the glabellar flap and created another nasal cutaneous flap that can be used for the nasal tip and midnasal wounds and called it the "dorsal nasal flap." The entire dorsal nasal skin, including a triangular glabellar extension is elevated and pivoted caudally.[5,9] In 1984, Marchac and Toth[10] modified Rieger's flap by narrowing the pedicle and creating an axial flap based on the blood supply that emerging from the medial canthus. This allowed a radical sliding and rotation of the frontonasal flap. Rohrich used it without a glabellar incision.[5,10,11]

Anatomy

Knowledge of the blood supply of the forehead, nasal, and paranasal region is paramount for the glabellar flap design (Fig. 1). The supratrochlear and supraorbital arteries, arising from the internal carotid artery, provides the blood supply to the forehead, glabellar, and medial canthal areas. The dorsum, lateral walls, and surface of the nose are supplied by an extensive branching network between the angular artery (terminal branch from the facial artery) and the dorsal nasal artery (which arises from the ophthalmic artery). The dorsal nasal artery pierces the orbital septum above the medial palpebral ligament and travels along the side of the nose to anastomose with the angular artery through the lateral nasal artery. The dorsal nasal artery provides a rich axial blood

[a] Ascension-St. John Hospital, 11900 E 12 Mile Road, Suite 210, Warren, MI 48093, USA
[b] Head and Neck Oncology/Microvascular Surgery, Ascension-St. John Hospital, Detroit, MI, USA
[c] Oral/Maxillofacial Surgery, Ascension-St. John Hospital, 11900 E 12 MIle Road, Warren, MI 48093 USA
[d] Microvascular Surgery, Ascension-St. John Hospital, Detroit, MI, USA
* Corresponding author. Oral/Maxillofacial Surgery, Ascension-St. John Hospital, 11900 E 12 MIle Road, Warren, MI 48093.
E-mail address: carlos.ramirez@ascension.org

Atlas Oral Maxillofacial Surg Clin N Am 28 (2020) 43–48
1061-3315/20/© 2019 Elsevier Inc. All rights reserved.
https://doi.org/10.1016/j.cxom.2019.11.004

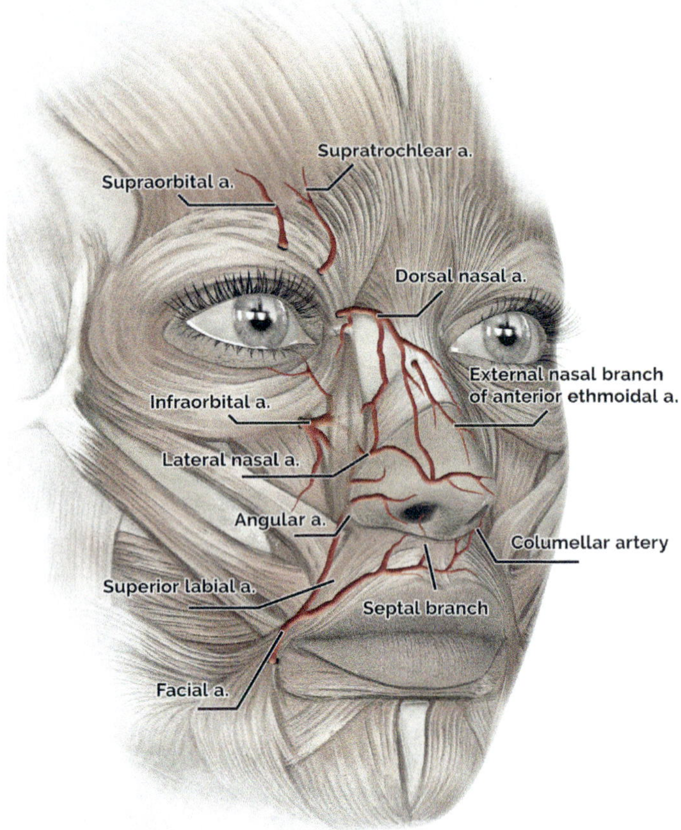

Fig. 1 Vascular supply of the nasal area.

supply to the dorsal nasal skin and serves as the main arterial contributor to the dorsal nasal flap.[2,5]

Four layers compose the soft tissue between the skin and the bony cartilaginous skeleton of the nose: (1) the superficial fatty layer, (2) the fibromuscular layer, (3) the deep fatty layer, and (4) the periosteum/perichondrium.[12] The skin of the glabella, nasal tip, and alae is thick and rigid owing to a thick fibromuscular layer and an abundant presence of sebaceous glands. On the other hand, the skin of the dorsum and sidewall is thin, smooth, and mobile.[2,5,13]

Indications

1. Reconstruction of defects in the middle and upper third of the nasal dorsum.
2. Reconstruction of the medial canthal area.
3. Reconstruction of middle and proximal nasal dorsum or tip of the nose, extending the traditional glabellar flap to form the dorsal nasal flap or frontonasal flap.

Surgical technique

Preoperative planning

Nasal defects are classified according to size, anatomic location, and depth. According to the subunit principle, if more than 50% of a subunit is involved, excision of the entire subunit before reconstruction is recommended.[1,13] However, many authors recommend using the subunit principle as a tool that should be modified to fit the individual needs of the patient, and not a rigid rule.[11,13]

Many flaps are described for nasal reconstruction; however, most defects can be closed with the dorsal nasal flap, glabellar flap, bilobe flap, V-Y advancement flap, nasolabial flap, or paramedian forehead flap, with the paramedian forehead flap being used for the most complex reconstructions.[13,14] Defects up to 1 cm in the cephalic two-thirds of the nose could be repaired primarily. The more cephalic it is, the easier the primary closure. The orientation of the reconstruction (vertical or horizontal) depends on the configuration of the defect and the degree of skin laxity.[5]

Preparation and patient positioning

Surgery can be done under local or general anesthesia depending on the planning, medical comorbidities, and patient and surgeon preference.

Surgical procedure

Glabellar flap for nasal reconstruction

Glabellar flap can be raised as a V-Y advancement flap, transposition flap, or a V-Y rotation advancement flap depending on the defect size and location.

V-Y advancement flap

- *Outlining the flap.* Locate the apex of the inverted V in the midpoint of glabellar region above the brow (Fig. 2). The first arm of the V passes superomedially from the defect toward the apex across the medial brow. The second arm arises from the apex and passes inferiorly to the other site of the defect.
- *Raising the flap.* The outlined skin and subcutaneous tissue are incised deep to the dermis into the subcutaneous fat. The adjacent tissue is undermined on both sides of the V in the same depth of the flap.
- *Flap insertion.* Mobility of the flap is checked to confirm the flap will reach the defect site without tension. The flap is advanced inferiorly to close the defect. The flap can be contoured at this time to fit the defect. The flap is inset with buried, interrupted, subcutaneous 3-0 or 4-0 Vicryl sutures.
- *Closure.* The skin is then closed with interrupted 5-0 or 6-0 nylon or Prolene sutures. The donor site is sutured in a V-Y closure, which may cause narrowing of the interbrow distance.

V-Y transposition and V-Y advancement rotation flap

- *Outlining the flap.* The apex of the V inverted is located in the same axis as the glabellar midpoint (Fig. 3). When rotation is needed, both segments of the flap should extend below the brow. The first arm arises from the defect to the apex superomedially. The length of the first arm of the V is important and should be longer, because this part must correspond with the most inferior margin of the defect. The second arm arises from the apex of the V and passes inferiorly to the other site of the defect at an usually at an angle of 45° and always less than 60°.
- *Raising the flap.* The outlined skin and subcutaneous tissue are incised to the level deep to the dermis and the adjacent skin is undermined extensively in the

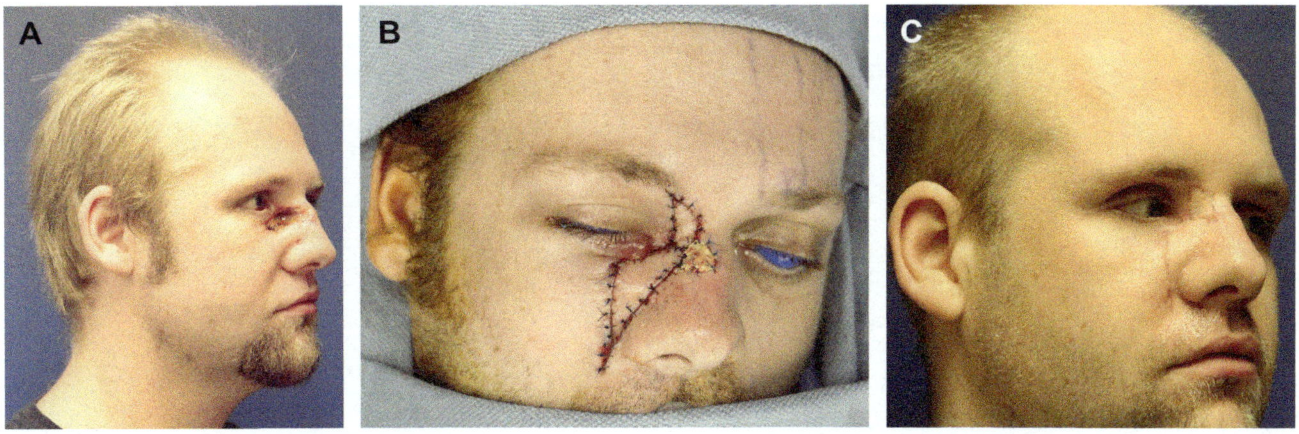

Fig. 2 Glabellar variant V-Y advancement flap. (*A*) Medial canthal defect. (*B*) Double V-Y advancement. (*C*) Double V-Y advancement flap for canthal reconstruction 3 months after surgery.

subcutaneous plane. Thinning of the subcutaneous fat can be done at this point if there is a discrepancy in thickness.

- *Flap insertion*. The flap is rotated inferomedially. The first arm with its apex is placed at the inferior tip of the defect, correcting the vertical height. The tip of the flap is trimmed to fit the defect and the flap is secured with buried, interrupted, subcutaneous 3-0 or 4-0 Vicryl sutures.
- *Closure*. Closure begins in a vertical fashion to create a V-Y pattern with the undermined tissue margins at the donor

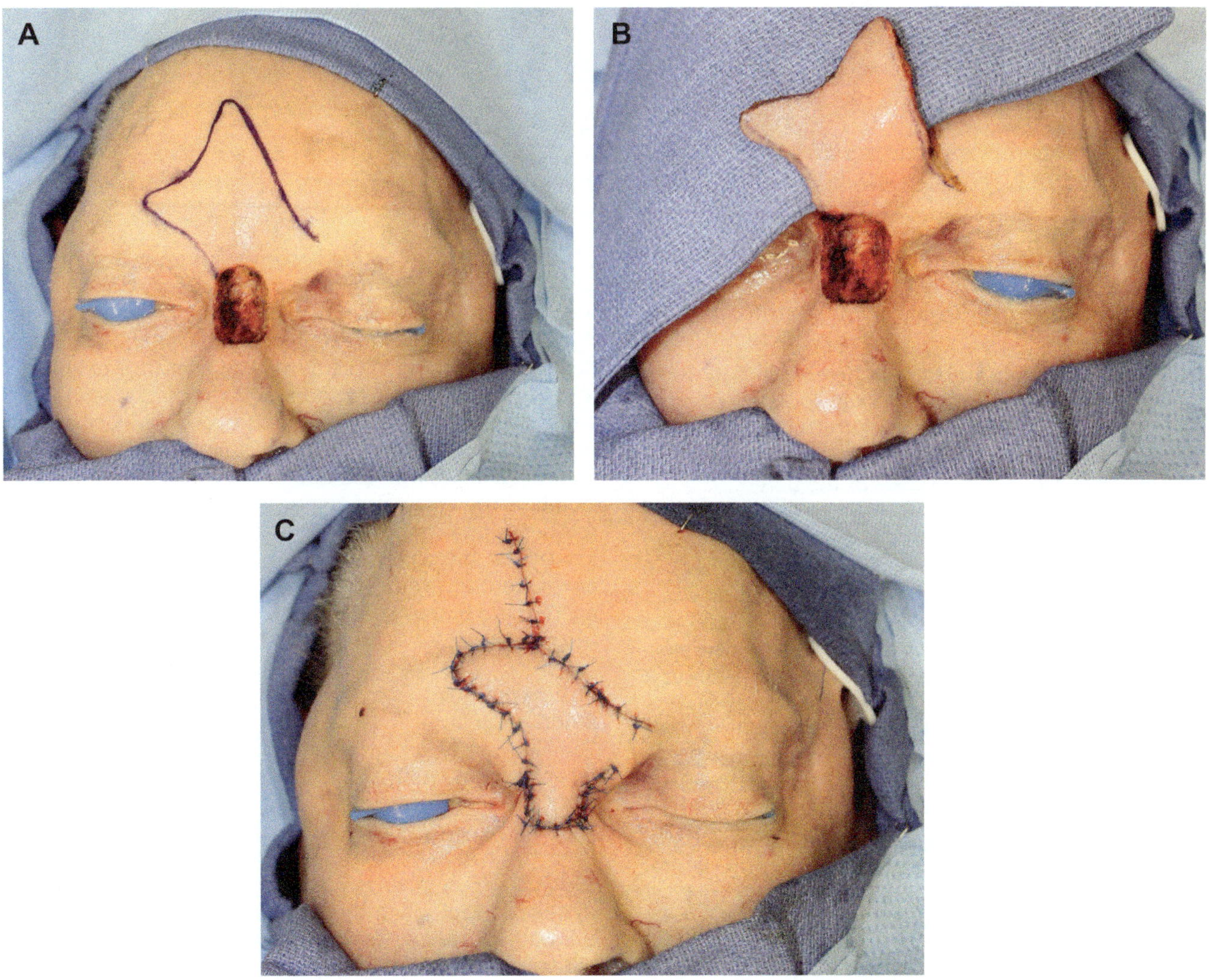

Fig. 3 Glabellar V-Y rotation flap. (*A*) Defect and flap markings. (*B*) Flap elevation and undermining. (*C*) Flap inset. (*Courtesy of* Rui P. Fernandes, MD, DMD, FACS, FRCS(Ed), Jacksonville, FL.)

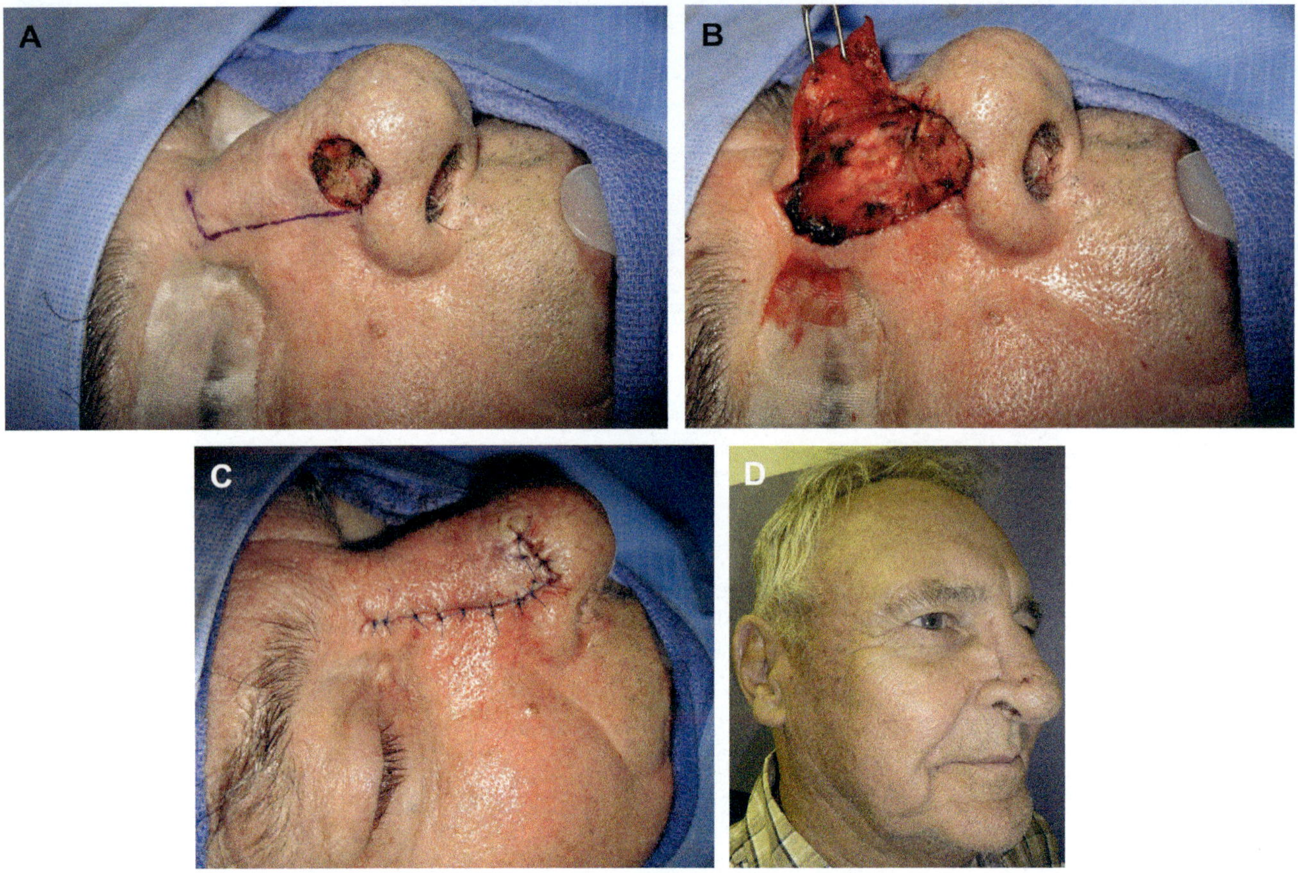

Fig. 4 Dorsal nasal flap. (*A*) Defect and flap design markings. (*B*) Dorsal nasal flap elevation. (*C*) Flap inset and closure. (*D*) Postoperative healing. (*Courtesy of* Rui P. Fernandes, MD, DMD, FACS, FRCS(Ed), Jacksonville, FL.)

site. Once the vertical closure is complete, the remaining defect is closed during flap inset. The skin is then closed with interrupted 5-0 or 6-0 nylon or Prolene sutures.

Dorsal nasal flap, frontonasal flap, and heminasal flap
The dorsal nasal flap can be based on a random supply (Rieger) or an axial supply from the angular or infratrochlear arteries (Marchac) (Figs. 4 and 5). The latter is designed with the pedicle arising from the ipsilateral side of the defect.[9,10]

- *Outlining the flap*. The outlined skin starts from an inverted V incision into the glabellar area. The second arm of the V extends inferiorly along the lateral nasal wall. An alternative could be done as an heminasal flap (see Fig. 5) with inferior extension of the flap traversing directly in the midline of the nose and preserving a lateral base along the nasal facial sulcus.
- *Raising the flap*. The outlined skin is incised with electrocautery and undermined extensively in a submuscular plane.
- *Flap insertion*. The flap is pivoted and rotated caudally into place. The flap is contoured to fit the defect. The standing cutaneous deformity is excised as needed. To ease closure, undermining the nasal tip and the lateral nasal side is completed.
- *Closure*. The donor site is closed in a V-Y fashion in the glabellar region. The flap is sutured in place using buried, interrupted, subcutaneous 3-0 or 4-0 sutures. The skin is then closed with interrupted 5-0 or 6-0 nylon or Prolene sutures.

Glabellar flap for canthal reconstruction
Reconstruction of canthal defects is challenging and can be done with multiple procedures including the glabellar V-Y advancement rotational flap or the bilobed flap (see Fig. 2). Flap design depends on the size of the defect, the distance to glabellar region, and the contour and depth of the medial canthus.[2,5] Patients with a flat nasal bridge and short nose will need a smaller flap than those with more prominent features. Regarding the V-Y flap, differences with the traditional glabellar flap in the height of the V, the angulation between the 2 arms of the V and the relationship of the V to the defect will depend on the size and location of the defect. The V is classically described as being placed centrally within the glabellar region, but it could be more appropriate to displace the apex to the side of the defect when reconstructing the canthal region.[4]

Alternative flaps from the glabellar region
Rintala flap
This flap can be an alternative for mid nasal supra-tip and tip reconstruction. As a random pattern flap, the length of the flap is its greatest disadvantage. The flap should be outlined with bilateral parallel incisions on both sides of the nasal sidewalls from the corner of the defect with extension into glabellar region.[15,16] The flap is elevated in a supraperichondral and supraperiosteal plane in the glabellar region. To allow sufficient advancement, Burow's triangles are excised bilaterally at the base of flap, typically above the level of the eyebrows to avoid their displacement. If necessary, when the flap advancement is short, they can be performed below the

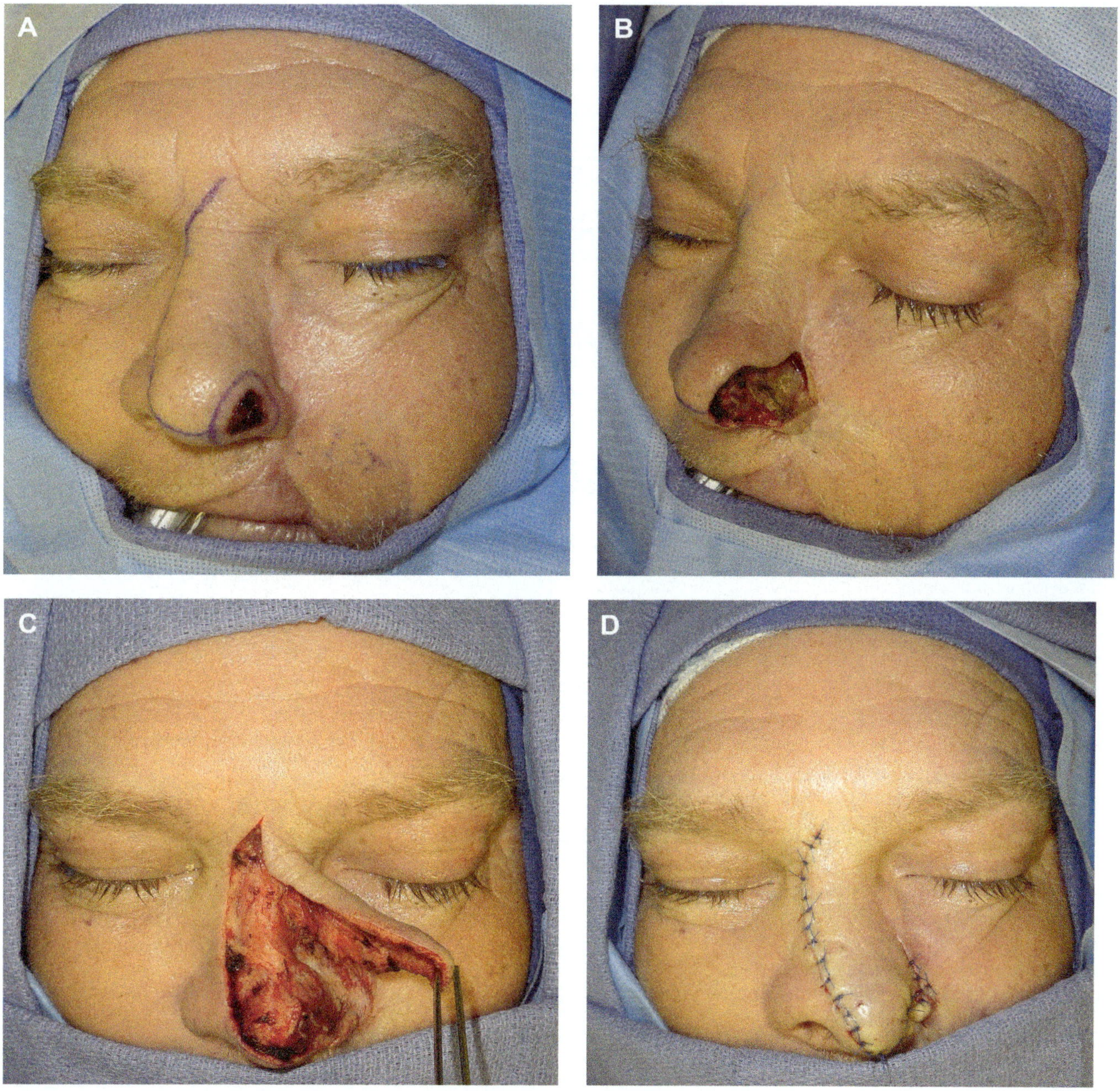

Fig. 5 Heminasal flap. (*A*) Preoperative flap markings. (*B*) Defect created. (*C*) Heminasal flap elevation. (*D*) Flap inset and closure. (*Courtesy of* Rui P. Fernandes, MD, DMD, FACS, FRCS(Ed), Jacksonville, FL.)

eyebrows.[17] The flap is sutured in place using buried, interrupted, subcutaneous 3-0 or 4-0 sutures. The skin is then closed with interrupted 5-0 or 6-0 nylon or Prolene sutures.

Island flap

Reverse island flaps from the glabellar and canthal region have been described for reconstruction of nasal tip, alae and upper lip. These flaps are based on terminal branches of facial vessels, which should be located and marked.[3] Templates of the defect can be used to outline the flap design in glabellar or canthal area. The incision should extend inferiorly along the nasal cheek junction toward the alar groove. Flaps should be raised in a supraperiosteal plane with a soft tissue cuff around the pedicle. Care must be taken when dissecting the pedicle superiorly because it is closely adherent to the periosteum. The donor site can be typically closed primarily, using a skin graft or with local advancement or transposition flaps.[6]

Potential complications

1. Noticeable scaring.
2. Lymphedema of flap tip, usually maximal at 3 months.
3. Necrosis of the tip and edges of flap in the early postoperative period, especially if the dissection is too superficial.
4. Thickening of the inferior margin of the flap requiring late debulking.
5. Widening of the limbus owing to tension on the medial canthus and unwanted pull on the medially situated brow areas.

Pearls and pitfalls

The glabellar flap can be easily performed using local skin that is of similar structure, texture, consistency, and color to that of the defect. The donor site defect can be closed primarily in most cases, and the incisions and resultant scars are generally well-camouflaged.[18,19] However, closure of the donor-site defect can lead to narrowing of the interbrow distance.[2,19]

Skin thickness between the glabella and other subunits is frequently discrepant.[4] To overcome this thickness discrepancy, the flap may be thinned significantly at the time of harvest by resecting of most of subcutaneous fatty tissues in approximately one-half of the distal side of the flap. This is possible because of the stable subcutaneous vascular network of the lateral nose provided by the angular artery and the dorsal nasal artery.[2]

Convexities and concavities of this area and the varying planes should be considered before the design of the flap.[8] Dorsal nasal flap has the disadvantage of causing juxtaposition of thick skin from the glabella to thin skin of the medial canthus. The dorsal heminasal flap avoids this disadvantage by maintaining the thin skin of the cephalic nasal sidewall. Another common disadvantage of the dorsal nasal flap is the cephalic rotation of the nostril margins and nasal tip, which may occur when the incisions are extended too far superiorly into the glabella.[2] This could be beneficial in case of tip ptosis in elder patients, but unacceptable in younger ones.[5] Marchac's modification of narrowing the pedicle has been described to help prevent nostril elevation.[10]

Immediate postoperative care

The patient is instructed to apply a thin layer of antibiotic ointment and remove crusting. The area is kept dry for 48 hours. Sutures are removed in 5 to 7 days to minimize scarring and redressed with adhesive bandage such as Steri-strips and left in place for an additional 48 to 72 hours.

Rehabilitation and recovery

No special postoperative rehabilitation is needed. The authors of this article and previous series published reported cosmetically acceptable results with no signs of functional deficit with this flap.

Summary

The glabellar area is a resource of redundant and thick skin and is used for the reconstruction of the upper nasal dorsum or medial canthal area. It provides local skin that is of similar structure, texture, consistency, and color to that of the defect. Glabellar flap can be modified or use in combination with other procedures to reconstruct more distal defects. It can be performed as a V-Y advancement flap, transposition flap or a V-Y rotation advancement flap regarding the defect size and location. Although scar is commonly well-camouflaged, potential scar and skin thickness differences between the glabella and other subunits may happen. To overcome this, the flap may be thinned significantly at the time of harvest.

Disclosure

The authors have nothing to disclose.

References

1. Burget GC, Menick F. The subunit principle in nasal reconstruction. Plast Reconstr Surg 1985;76:239e47.
2. Koch CA, Archibald DJ, Friedman O. Glabellar flaps in nasal reconstruction. Facial Plast Surg Clin North Am 2011;19(1):113–22.
3. Asaria J, Pepper JP, Baker SR. Key issues in nasal reconstruction. Curr Opin Otolaryngol Head Neck Surg 2010;18(4):278–82.
4. Maloof AJ, Leatherbarrow B. The glabellar flap dissected. Eye 2000;14(4):597–605.
5. Baker SR. Principles of nasal reconstruction. New York: Springer; 2011.
6. Morrison WA, Donato RR, Breidahl AF, et al. Island inner canthal and glabellar flaps for nasal tip reconstruction. Br J Plast Surg 1995;48(5):263–70.
7. Seyhan T. The radix nasi island flap. J Craniofac Surg 2009;20(2): 516–21.
8. Field LM. The glabellar transposition " Banner " Flap. J Dermatolog Surg Oncol 1988;14(4):376–9.
9. Rieger RA. A local flap for repair of the nasal tip. Plast Reconstr Surg 1967;40(2):147–9.
10. Marchac D, Toth B. The axial frontonasal flap revisited. Plast Reconstr Surg 1985;76(5):686–94.
11. Rohrich RJ, Muzaffar AR, Adams WP Jr. The aesthetic unit dorsal nasal flap: rationale for avoiding a glabellar incision. Plast Reconstr Surg 1999;104:1289–94.
12. Oneal RM, Beil RJ. Surgical anatomy of the nose. Adv Aesthetic Rhinoplasty Art, Sci New Clin Tech 2013;37(2):33–60.
13. Parrett BM, Pribaz JJ. An algorithm for treatment of nasal defects. Clin Plast Surg 2009;36(3):407–20.
14. Colletti G. Lemmo's flap for nasal dorsum reconstruction. J Oral Maxillofac Surg 2012;70(3):672–6.
15. Rintala AE, Asko-Seljavaara S. Reconstruction of midline skin defects of the nose. Scand J Plast Reconstr Surg 1969;3:105–8.
16. Ebrahimi A, Nejadsarvari N, Koushki ES. Application of modified Rintala flap in nasal tip reconstruction. Am J Otolaryngol 2012; 33(6):685–8.
17. Onishi K, Okada E, Hirata A. The Rintala flap: a versatile procedure for nasal reconstruction. Am J Otolaryngol 2014;35(5):577–81.
18. Uzun H, Bitik O, Kamburoğlu HO, et al. Assessment of patients who underwent nasal reconstruction after non-melanoma skin cancer excision. J Craniofac Surg 2015;26(4):1299–303.
19. Konofaos P, Alvarez S, McKinnie JE, et al. Nasal reconstruction: a simplified approach based on 419 operated cases. Aesthetic Plast Surg 2015;39(1):91–9.

Bilobed Flaps

Cong Vo, DDS, MD [a], William Walsh Thomas, MD [b], Hans C. Brockhoff II, DDS, MD [c], Daniel Petrisor, DMD, MD [a,*]

KEYWORDS

• Bilobed flap • Skin cancer • Local defect reconstruction • Facial reconstruction • Nasal reconstruction

KEY POINTS

- Bilobed flaps are excellent local reconstructive options for nasal dorsum, tip, and sidewall defects.
- The bilobed flap can be applied to other areas of the face and enlarged considerably because it is similar in concept to the cervicofacial advancement flap.
- Wide undermining of adjacent skin, thinning of the flap at the initial inset, and use of angled incisions can help minimize the incidence and severity of a trapdoor deformity.

Introduction

Local tissue rearrangement and flap reconstruction of the head and neck have a long and storied history. Much interest has been placed on selecting and executing the appropriate flap to reconstruct an ablative defect. Bilobed flaps are among the many techniques available to a surgeon. They are double transposition flaps that share a single base. The flaps move around pivotal points located at the base. This naturally creates a standing cutaneous deformity and a reduction in length as the flap pivots.[1] Most often these flaps are random cutaneous and thus subjected to the restrictive parameters (length-to-width ratios) required by this type of flap.

Historically, the first description of a bilobed flap was in 1918. Esser[2] described the pedicled bilobed flap for nasal tip reconstruction, which draws on tissue that is adjacent to the skin defect, allowing for excellent texture and color match. Esser described a double transposition of 2 equal-sized flaps with a 180o total arc of rotation, which ultimately harvested skin from the glabellar region.[2] The tension from such a large arc of rotation, however, increased the risk of flap necrosis and created unwanted cosmetic outcomes, such as dog-ears and pin-cushioning. Subsequently, several modifications have been described in the literature that aimed to minimize these complications. In 1953, Zimany modified the flap to use successively smaller lobes, allowing for a more esthetic closure without excessive tissue harvesting.[3] In 1989, Zitelli[4] decreased the total rotational arc to 90° to 100°. The smaller rotational arc helps to reduce tension, which improved the cosmetic result. This is the modification used most often today.[4] Application of the bilobed flap has expanded beyond nasal reconstruction to include repair of other locations in the face like the cheek, ear, upper lip, zygoma, and orbit.[5–7]

Bilobed flaps for smaller-sized defects have shown acceptable esthetic outcomes and low rates of complications. Salgarelli and colleagues[8] reported their experience with the use of 285 consecutive Zitelli bilobed flaps used for facial reconstruction of various sites. They examined these flaps after the resection of basal cell carcinomas or squamous cell carcinomas, with defect sizes between 1 cm and 4 cm. They reported a 3.6% postoperative complication rate, with 2 cases of local infection, 1 complete flap necrosis, and 7 cases of partial necrosis requiring partial revision.[8]

Although bilobed flaps traditionally have been utilized for smaller reconstructive defects around the face and neck, Mourad and colleagues[9] demonstrated their utility in reconstruction of various larger defects. A total of 23 giant bilobed flaps were used, with the average-sized defect 27.2 cm. All closures were achieved in a single stage without the need for tissue expanders, free tissue transfers, or skin grafts. They reported acceptable cosmetic outcomes with no wound complications or flap breakdowns. In these cases, the bilobed flap functions much like a very large cervicofacial advancement flap because skin laxity from the neck and even chest can function as a double transposition flap with primary closure of the donor site. Moore and colleagues[10] illustrated the great versatility of local double transposition flaps for large head and neck defects in a 33 patient series. Although limited by the small number of the series, the investigators found no detrimental impact of prior smoking, prior radiation, or medical comorbidities, illustrating the robust nature of these flaps and their applications for patients unfit for free tissue transfer.

Nasal anatomy

The nose can be divided into 3 zones, each with different tissue characteristics.[11] Zone 1 includes the upper half the nose and is made of thin, movable tissue. Zone 2, which includes the ala and tip, is made of skin that is sebaceous, thick, and less movable. Zone 3 has tissue characteristics that are similar to those of zone 1 and includes the columella and infratip lobule.

[a] OHSU Oral & Maxillofacial Surgery Clinic, Mark O. Hatfield Research Center, 3250 SW Sam Jackson Park Road, Portland, OR 97239, USA
[b] 3485 SW Bond Avenue, Building 2, 9th Floor, Portland, OR 97239, USA
[c] 0175 Gateway Blvd W Suite 304, El Paso, TX 79925, USA
* Corresponding author.
E-mail address: petrisor@ohsu.edu

Atlas Oral Maxillofacial Surg Clin N Am 28 (2020) 49–52
1061-3315/20/Published by Elsevier Inc.
https://doi.org/10.1016/j.cxom.2019.11.002

There is a rich blood supply to the skin of the nose that comes laterally via tributaries of the angular artery and from the columellar artery as a branch of the superior labial artery. The dorsal nasal artery and infraorbital artery also contribute to the vascular supply of the nose and have multiple anastomoses, with the branches of the angular artery giving the nose a rich blood supply for local flap reconstruction.[12]

Surgical technique

See Figs. 1–3.

- Circumscribe the skin defect in a circular fashion.
- Note the center of the defect and measure the radius, "r".
- Next, determine the pivot point, also known as the base. The pivot point is marked 1r length, perpendicularly from the edge of the defect, typically placed lateral to the defect. The region approximately 90° from the lesion about this pivot point should be an area with sufficient tissue laxity to accommodate transposition.
- Mark a line from the pivot point that is 90° - 110° to the line created between center of the lesion and the pivot point. The angle created is the total axis of rotation for the entire flap.
- To plan for the donor site design, 2 concentric 90° arcs are drawn with the pivot point as the center.
- The first arc is drawn 2r from the pivot point, and the second arc is drawn 3r from the pivot.

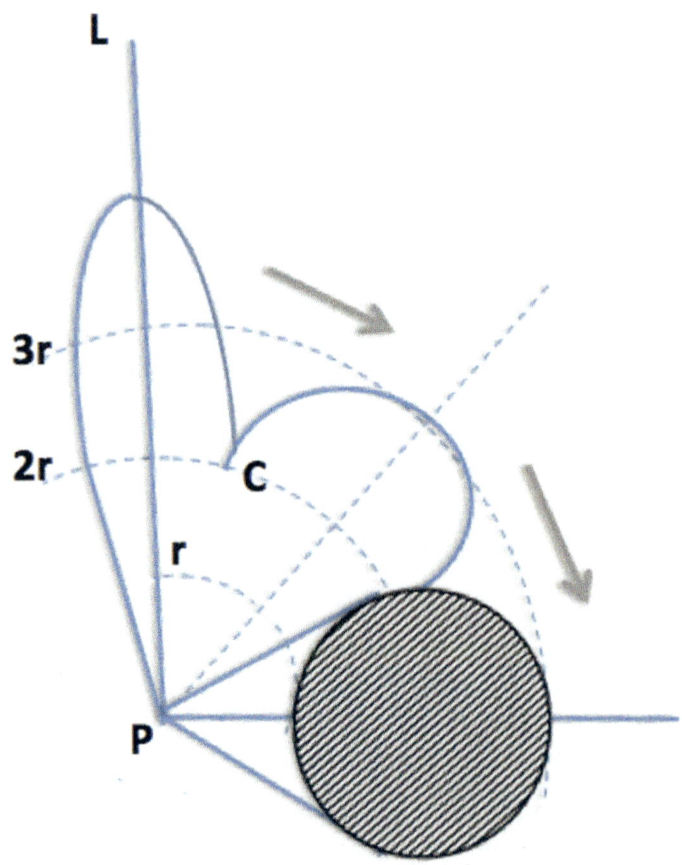

Fig. 1 Design of the bilobed flap. C, corner between first and second lobes; L, line drawn from the pivot point (P) that is 90° - 110° to the line created between center of the defect and P.

- The first lobe, that is, the primary donor site, is drawn as a circle adjacent to the defect, with its center 45° from the center of the lesion, about the pivot point (P). The width of this circle should be approximately equal to the width of the defect, but no bigger. As such, the radius of this lobe is 1r and should reach the outermost arc. In tissues with more laxity than nasal skin, the width of primary donor site can be 1/2r of the defect because undermining allows closure of the wound.
- The second lobe is approximately triangular in shape, with its center 45° from the center of the first lobe. The second lobe is drawn adjacent to the first lobe, with its base corner at the previously drawn inner arch, adjacent to the base of the first donor site. The width of the base should be slightly smaller than the width of defect. The apex of this triangle should extend just beyond the outer arc to complete the outline of the bilobed flap.
- To allow for rotation of the flap into the defect, draw 2 tangent lines from the pivot point to the skin defect. The resulting V-shaped tracing (also known as the Burow triangle) is excised to allow for rotation of the flap.
- The flaps are elevated in a supra-perichondrial plane.
- The surrounding tissue is elevated in a supra-periosteal and supra-perichondrial plane or in a submuscular plane in laterally based flaps.
- Remember that the thickness of the transposed flap depends on the depth of the defect. As such, the subcutaneous tissues should be trimmed accordingly.
- The terminal donor site is closed primarily.
- The lobules are inset with deep, 5-0 absorbable monofilament sutures in a horizontal mattress technique, and the skin is closed with meticulous care in the surgeon's preferred method.

Modifications

Since Zitelli, several investigators have described additional variations to the bilobed flap. Although the flap is commonly laterally based to take advantage the rich blood supply to the nose, the literature has described medially and superiorly based flaps. Kelly-Sell and colleagues[13] described a superiorly based flap where the terminal donor site closure is continuous with the mesiolabial fold, creating an esthetic closure. Wang and colleagues[14] used a technique that draws from the laxity of adjacent tissue of the cheek, allowing for harvest of greater quantities of tissue. The trilobe flap uses the same principles as the bilobed flap, adding a third donor site that allows for more versatility.[15] Using this technique, the surgeon can access tissue from a more distant reservoir or place the closure of the terminal donor site in an esthetic area.

Pearls and pitfalls

Advantages

1. Harvesting of adjacent skin, which allows for excellent tissue match; avoiding depressions that are common with skin grafts
2. Single-stage procedure with thinning of the flap done at time of insetting
3. Low morbidity, predictable tissue viability

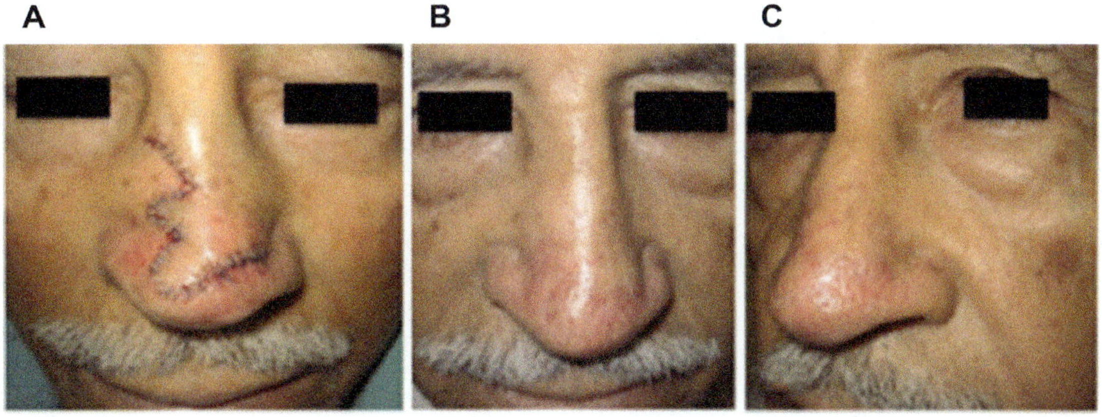

Fig. 2 (*A*) Superiorly based bilobed flap of the dorsum and nasal tip. Frontal (*B*) and 3/4-view (*C*), postoperative images illustrate excellent healing of the donor scars as well as no trapdoor deformity. Nasal alar margins and tip are unchanged with this reconstruction.

Limitations

1. Risk of retraction in alar defects and defect close to the nasal margin
2. Poor lymphatic drainage from superiorly based flaps
3. Thick skin, additional skin lesions, or other defects at site of proposed flap

Potential complications

Due to the unique anatomic characteristics of the caudal nose, undesirable cosmetic outcomes can occur.[16,17] When defects are close to the nasal margin, wound tension and contraction can cause distortion of the nasal tip, pulling it upward. Furthermore, there is a tendency for the transposed tissue to appear more

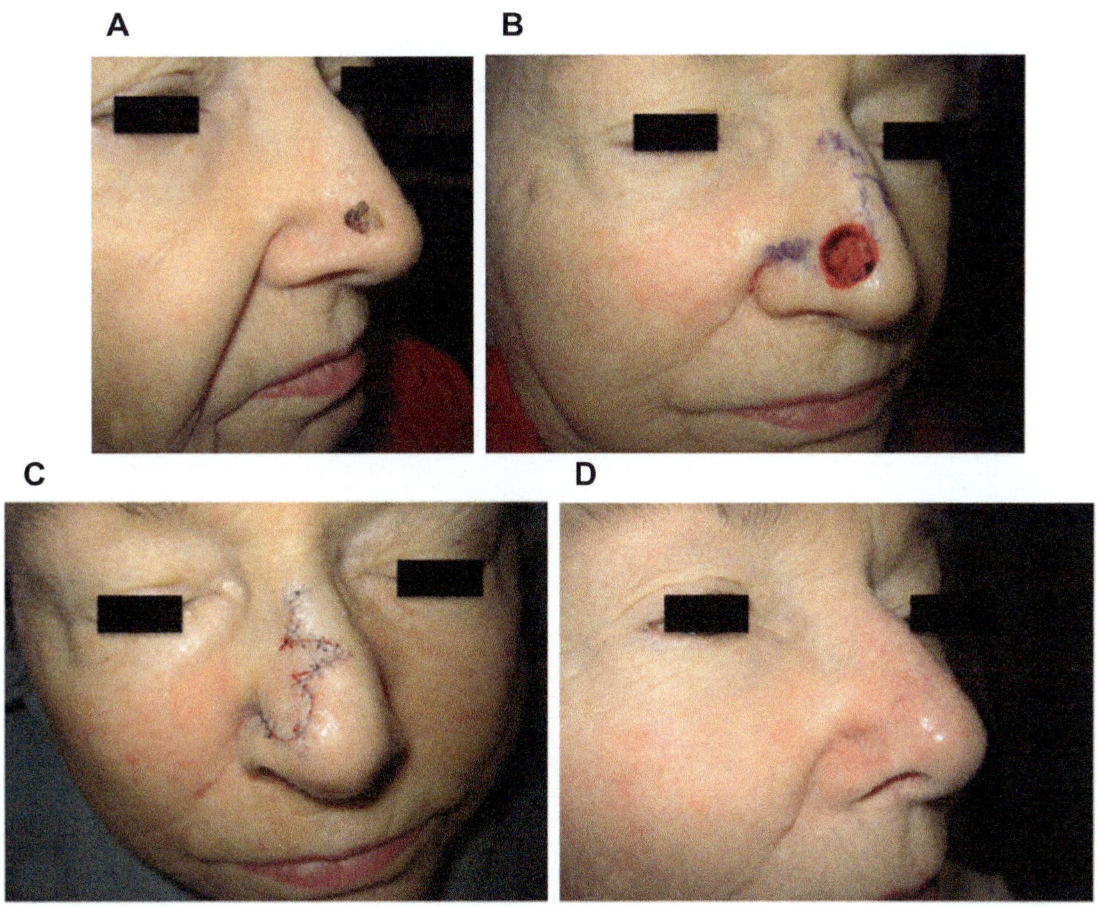

Fig. 3 (*A*) A 68-year-old woman with squamous cell carcinoma of the right lateral nose. (*B*) Postablative surgical defect. (*C*) Bilobed flap elevated and inset into defect. (*D*) Bilobed flap displays good color match and tissue thickness at 3 months postoperatively.

elevated or puffy than the surrounding tissues, also known as a trapdoor deformity or pin-cushioning. This typically becomes evident approximately 3 months postoperatively. This type of deformity can be avoided or minimized by sufficiently undermining the tissues surrounding the donor site and ablative defect during time of flap harvest and insetting. If pin-cushioning does occur, it can be managed with triamcinolone acetonide injections. If surgical revision is necessary, the trapdoor deformity can be excised and the adjacent tissue reapproximated after adequate undermining. In rare cases of insufficient nasal tip support, nasal obstruction can occur. Typically, this can be corrected only with surgical repair of the external and/or internal nasal valves. Additionally, unsightly or widened scars can be an indication for dermabrasion in the postoperative period (6–8 weeks) or any time during scar maturation (1 year). The donor site scar, flap, and entire nasal subunit are dermabraded to pinpoint bleeding, and the adjacent tissue to the subunit is lightly dermabraded to blend the transition.

Summary

The bilobed flap is a versatile, reliable local flap that achieves excellent esthetic results. It is a technique that reconstructive surgeons should have in their repertoire of reconstruction modalities for not only nasal but also facial skin defects. Although the flap typically is a single-stage procedure, there occasionally may be a need for minor revisions in the postoperative period.

Disclosure

The authors have nothing to disclose.

References

1. Baker S. Local flaps in facial reconstruction. 3rd edition. Philadelphia: Saunders; 2014.
2. Esser J. Gestielte Lokale Nasenplastik Mit Zweizipfligem Lappen, Deckung Des Sekundären Defektes Vom Ersten Zipfel Durch Den Zweiten. Deutsche Zeitschrift Für Chirurgie 1918;143(3–6):385–90.
3. Zimany A. The bilobed flap. Plast Reconstr Surg 1953;11(6):424–34.
4. Zitelli J. The bilobed flap for nasal reconstruction. Arch Dermatol 1989;125(7):957–9.
5. Blige A, Yazici B, Kasapoglu F. Reconstruction of orbital exenteration defects with bilobed forehead flaps. Int Ophthalmol 2016;36(6):861–5.
6. White CP, Rosen N, Muhn CY. The usefulness of the bilobed flap for lateral cheek defects. Can J Plast Surg 2012;20(1):e19–21.
7. Mutaf M, Isk D, Atik B, et al. Versatility of the bilobed cervical skin flap for total ear reconstruction in the unfavorable temporoauriculomastoid region. Plast Reconstr Surg 2006;118(3):652–62.
8. Salgarelli A, Cangiano A, Sartorelli F, et al. The bilobed flap in skin cancer of the face: our experience on 285 cases. J Craniomaxillofac Surg 2010;38(6):460–4.
9. Mourad M, Arnaoutakis D, Sawhney R, et al. Use of giant bilobed flap for advanced head and neck defects. Facial Plast Surg 2016;32(3):320–4.
10. Moore B, Wine T, Netterville J. Cervicofacial and cervicothoracic rotation flaps in head and neck reconstruction. Head Neck 2005;27(12):1092–101.
11. Burget G, Menick F. Aesthetic reconstruction of the nose. 2nd edition. St Louis (MO): Mosby; 1994.
12. Pilsl U, Anderhuber F. The external nose: the nasal arteries and their course in relation to the nasolabial fold and groove. Plast Reconstr Surg 2016;138(5):830–5.
13. Kelly-Sell M, Hollmi S, Cook J. The superiorly based bilobed flap for nasal reconstruction. J Am Acad Dermatol 2018;78(2):370–6.
14. Wang Z, Chen X, Chen Z. A modified bilobed flap design for nasal tip defects. Plast Aesthet Res 2014;1:16–20.
15. Albertini J, Hansen J. Trilobed flap reconstruction for distal nasal skin defects. Dermatol Surg 2010;36(11):1726–35.
16. Steiger J. Bilobed flaps in nasal reconstruction. Facial Plast Surg Clin North Am 2011;19(1):107–11.
17. Baker S. Principles of nasal reconstruction. 2nd edition. New York: Springer; 2011.

Moving?

Make sure your subscription moves with you!

To notify us of your new address, find your **Clinics Account Number** (located on your mailing label above your name), and contact customer service at:

Email: journalscustomerservice-usa@elsevier.com

800-654-2452 **(subscribers in the U.S. & Canada)**
314-447-8871 **(subscribers outside of the U.S. & Canada)**

Fax number: 314-447-8029

Elsevier Health Sciences Division
Subscription Customer Service
3251 Riverport Lane
Maryland Heights, MO 63043

*To ensure uninterrupted delivery of your subscription, please notify us at least 4 weeks in advance of move.

ELSEVIER

Sheridan
Hanover, PA USA
July 29, 2022